I0129670

Secrets About Back Pain And Fibromyalgia

How Common Back Pain Can Become Fibromyalgia

Sunny Kierstyn RN, DC

INTERNATIONAL HEALTH PUBLISHING

www.InternationalHealthPublishing.com

INTERNATIONAL HEALTH PUBLISHING
Founded February 2008
Publishing Group Affirming Truth & Innate Wisdom

For information about special discounts for bulk purchase, please contact International Health Publishing at writer@InternationalHealthPublishing.com.

International Health Publishing can bring authors to your live events. For more information or to book an event, contact writer@InternationalHealthPublishing.com or visit our website: www.InternationalHealthPublishing.com.

Secrets About Back Pain And Fibromyalgia
How Common Back Pain Can Become Fibromyalgia
Sunny Kierstyn RN, DC

First trade paperback edition October 2014
Copyright © 2013 by Sunny Kierstyn
Foreword copyright © 2013 by Sunny Kierstyn
SOT illustrations copyright © 2013 Dr. Jonathon Howat

Fibrocare.org

ISBN-13 978-0-9857956-2-7

ePUB ISBN-13 978-0-9857956-3-4

Library of Congress Control Number: 2012954406

SAN 856-6925

Manufactured in the United States of America, and printed on the finest 100% postconsumer-waste recycled paper

10 9 8 7 6 5 4 3 2 1

Gratitude

It took a MAJOR village to write this book.

This is one of those books where it took the entirety of my life to understand the complex in a simple manner. At least I hope it comes across as simple.

To get to this stage, there are so many people to whom I owe gratitude and a *GIANT Thank You*. An old saying I've heard more than once is so true: *"When the student is ready, the teacher will appear."* I have been so blessed with and by the teachers who crossed my path. Thank you and blessings to all of you!

To these wonderful people and groups, I owe a huge deal of gratitude...

To you, the wonderful doctors and teachers and professors who taught me chiropractic. I am honored and humbled to be able to do this incredible and health-promoting work.

To you, the people who, during my nursing career, allowed me to provide you healing services at your most vulnerable moments. Your courage gave me strength, taught me compassion and patience, and enhanced my understanding of the human body on daily basis. I will be forever grateful for your kindnesses.

To you, the wonderful people who, since my doctor-hood, have allowed me the honor of working with your bodies and physical challenges. Again and again, you've taught me to avoid underestimating what the human body can do and can achieve. You continue to teach me about the miraculous human body.

To you, my incredible Fibromyalgia patients: your courage and stoic-ness is a daily inspiration. Watching each of you breakthrough, regain your health, and begin to live again is one of the greatest joys in my life.

To you, my sister Colleen, who has been a precious guide all the time we've been allowed to be on this planet together.

To you, my wonderful children – and grandchildren – for your patience with my learning as I go through my career years.

To my college study partner, Dr. Howard Friedman, for finding Sacral Occipital Technique and making sure I didn't ignore it while we both still managed to get through microbiology class.

To you, my patient and forgiving peers, friends and family who so graciously volunteered to read the raw manuscript of this book, giving me guidance at a critical time in its evolution and providing your feedback.

To you: the American public, for your willingness to learn, to read this book and to realize the need for insights about your body beyond the current norm.

Starting with Dr. DeJarnette in the 1920s, this book has evolved through and from the minds of many brilliant people. Each of the teachers and patients who have blessed my universe throughout my life have – in their own way – aided the evolution of this understanding. I will forever be grateful for each of those contributions.

My sincere appreciation is extended to Dr. Jonathon Howat for sharing his excellent depictions and illustrations of the Sacral Occipital Syndrome. Their beautiful simplicity speaks to the power of their message. Disease development CAN be as simple as a distorted power supply!

Special thanks to the content editors: Linda McDaniels Schiltke, DC, Herb Friedman, DC, and Dr. Annette Simard, DC. And special thanks to the illustrators: Anthony Christensen, Cassandra Wanner, Kelly DeForrest, and Steven Zeller (graphic artist).

Contents

Secrets About Back Pain And Fibromyalgia

How Common Back Pain Can Become Fibromyalgia

Foreword

We posed a question: Could fibromyalgia develop from an accumulation of misalignment patterns? We asked ourselves: Since common structural patterns are renown for provoking random pains and stresses within the human body, could those difficulties escalate? Are the body's 'usual' patterns of misalignments enough to contribute to the growing list of diseases that are now being considered as 'part of the fibromyalgia overall picture'.

We know those diagnoses can be enhanced through breathing or eating or drinking various things, but are the underlying pulls and tugs around the body that develop as we grow and don't exercise or sit and stand in habitual patterns enough to provoke dysfunction of a part such as a complex joint or organ? Is that enough to lead to actual disease? What provokes all of the inflammation? Are there other forces at play or is chronic distortion of our nervous systems enough to enable the intermittent yet on-going and escalating problems of fibromyalgia?

The truths we uncovered through our next 15 years of research still astound us. Despite frequent efforts to challenge our findings, all we get are more well patients!

Step One

1

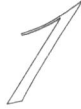

The Development of Fibromyalgia

The human body is absolutely exquisite: the way it automatically conducts itself through life, the way it repairs and recovers itself, the way it grows and develops itself innately.

To explain it simply would be an offense to our Creator. Yet with no offense to that Being, there is a level on which the human body is exquisitely simple. My hope for this book is to illustrate that simplicity, to you. From this simplicity grows the human's underlying, inherent structural and neurological strength.

This book is not intended to be an academic tome. It is written for you. Hopefully avoiding the majority of medicalese, its purpose is intended to offer mental pictures of how your body works, all together, synchronously, every day.

My intention is to illustrate the functions and dys-functions of the body using "word pictures," to create a three-dimensional mental and physical awareness about your body, and to allow you to think of your body in a way you may not have previously considered. You will discover how the body can 'go on tilt' as we live through our lives and visualize how that small yet profound 'tilt' can cause havoc and pain to the average human body. You will see how this can impact one's health (or the lack thereof) in an astounding way. This book illustrates how that little 'tilt' may ultimately lead to what we call 'fibromyalgia.'

That name fibromyalgia can send chills through people who suffer with this structural condition. They feel they can never get away from it. Our clinic has heard from many people who have felt this same way. What they found was that it IS possible to get away from it, to calm and quiet their body. In our approach, we 1.) address the condition as a skeletal structural condition, 2.) nourish the body to the point of cellular saturation, and 3.) eliminate (avoid) environmental substances known to provoke inflammation and cellular stress. By correcting structural imbalances, nourishing the body, and eliminating toxins, we witness people get out of pain, smile again, and even laugh and dance!

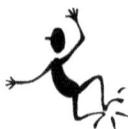

While never intending to come even close to claiming we are "curing" the fibromyalgia condition, our treatment plans, developed over the last dozen years, show strong signs of taming the problem. We routinely watch our patients get back into their lives!

In taming the symptoms of the fibromyalgia condition through the use of our recovery plans, we (the Fibromyalgia Care Center of Oregon) began to observe something we did not anticipate. We began to see that fibromyalgia sorted out into several types and we've identified several distinctive layers of severity as well. This book will teach you about three of the most important layers: 1.) the Chronic Sacroiliac Syndrome, 2.) Acquired ('Faux') Fibromyalgia and 3.) 'True' Fibromyalgia.

As our research developed, we began to notice a wider and wider division between Acquired Fibromyalgia and other types, enough to designate the general groups as 'faux' and 'true' fibromyalgia. Our growing graduate population of tamed 'faux' fibromyalgia patients – meaning those who had successfully worked through our treatment programs, stopped having structural or metabolic difficulties, and had returned fully to their lives – became more and more out of proportion compared to those who only slightly changed and lightened up, but did not fully improve to complete elimination of pain and irregular metabolic patterns.

Mind you, all of these were patients who arrived at the Fibromyalgia Care Center of Oregon *already diagnosed* by their MD with fibromyalgia. When we first welcomed them to our clinic, none had been designated with any particular *type* of fibromyalgia, but all had active trigger points enough to have been diagnosed with 'fibromyalgia.' Within *that* population we began seeing a division of people: one group corrected enough to be fully back within their lives – some within two weeks to ninety days – while others had difficulty with pain patterns which continued well beyond ninety days. The pain patterns and digestive concerns of the latter group would be tempered and improved but not totally freed from a periodic flare. 'True' Fibro patients can ultimately get back into their lives with our treatment plans, yet at times it has taken upwards of four to twelve months for them to be able to live their lives fully. And no, that previous statement was not a typo; I did say the majority "were corrected enough to be fully back within their lives within *two weeks to ninety days.*" They are the conditions we began to call the "Faux Fibro's."

'True' or 'Faux?'

The recovery time is the part we found so astounding! Some of the cases corrected so quickly and without complication that we believe they could only be part of a common skeletal configuration called the Chronic Sacroiliac Syndrome (CSS). CSS is a structural syndrome that generally affects most of the human population in varying degrees. It expresses itself with pelvic pain (in varying degrees) and low back discomfort, mid-back pain and anxiety, shoulder pain and neck pain, headaches and sinus problems, vertigo, knee problems and foot problems (like plantar fasciitis). It can be accompanied by indigestion, small bowel upsets, and heart palpitations... all very scary – and very real – symptoms. But these symptoms are also accompanied by sets of structural misalignments that create nerve and muscle problems. The misalignments arise out of using our bodies to live on the planet on a day-to-day basis; misalignments tend to accumulate and expand into other nearby joints as we move through life. It's important to recognize that all are *structural* problems, <u>not diseases</u>. And all can be corrected. Once misalignments are corrected, nerve physiology improves and the body stops experienc-

3

ing the symptoms that resulted from nerve interference. This simple principle is what I am hoping you will begin to understand. In addition, correcting dysfunction and misalignment in the body early on will enhance the recovery outcome to such a huge degree.

As I started writing this book about fibromyalgia, it didn't take long before realizing the need to define 'Faux' Fibromyalgia before being able to make sense of our discoveries with 'True' Fibromyalgia.

'Faux' Fibromyalgia

So, what do I mean when I say 'Faux Fibromyalgia? 'Faux' Fibromyalgia – or Acquired Fibromyalgia (as I am using it) – is another term for what is more commonly known as the Chronic Sacroiliac (Sak-ro-il-e-ak) Syndrome. An awkward term, the Chronic Sacroiliac Syndrome (CSS) describes a condition where a *group* of structural misalignments are found often accompanying one another. The group of misalignments reflects the involvement of body regions throughout the skeletal structure that become out of sync with one another. The misalignment patterns provoke the myriad of symptoms (some occurring constantly, some intermittently) that we often hear expressed from people diagnosed with fibromyalgia as their major points of concern and distress: pain around the eyes and around the head, pain at the base of the head or neck, tight shoulders, pain between or next to the shoulder blades, achy elbows, pain and tightness across the base of the spine, pain in the low back and at the sides of the upper legs, knees, ankles, with tender points developing at the shoulders and across the base of the skull or at the elbows, knees and in the low back, various types and degrees of organ dysfunction, etc. When the Chronic Sacroiliac Syndrome (CSS) flares-up or sounds-off with pain and/or dysfunction, the pain patterns strongly resemble what is being described as Fibromyalgia.

Teaching you to see this chain of connected nerve points is not in any way meant to demean, dismiss or invalidate the concerns these patients are feeling and expressing. You all ARE in pain! Every to every-other nerve relay station in their body is off center and screaming or groaning or stabbing at them. Teaching you this information is to open the understanding that chiropractic medicine has a solid understanding about this set of conditions.

A hundred percent of our already-diagnosed-as-fibromyalgia cases, we found, fit somewhere within this picture of the chronic sacroiliac syndrome... meaning their structural problems fit somewhere along its long arc of evolvement. Whether in the 'early' stage where ligaments weren't yet stretched, in the 'mild-moderate' stage where dysfunctional soft tissue patterns were beginning to develop but hadn't yet scarred and toughened into movement restrictions, or even the ones who HAD evolved into 'True' fibromyalgia patterns requiring greater focus: each of them presented with a structural condition that expressed some component of the Chronic Sacroiliac Syndrome. Through use of our multi-layered treatment plans, about 75% of patients were able to get back into their lives in a two week to ninety-day time span. This group of 75% we began to call 'Faux Fibro.' They present with the same types of symptoms and restrictions but seem to clear up – some almost entirely – within a short time, some just as quickly. That's the discussion within *this* book.

70% chronic sacroiliac syndrome: only needing treatment on an 'owie per owie' basis or between once per month and once per quarter; 30% fibromyalgia requiring a short treatment plan to bring under control and light maintenance schedule to keep it quiet with 10% 'True' Fibromyalgia requiring a more assertive/longer treatment plan and a longer stabilizing time period before it can stay quieted on a maintenance plan.

Trigger Points As Diagnostic Criteria

In 1989, the Academy of Rheumatology, a division within the American Medical Association, created the criteria of Trigger Points to be used as a method for the identification and diagnosis of fibromyalgia. When a person reaches the point where eleven of those standard eighteen trigger points are positive (or painful to a touch of a certain magnitude), a diagnosis of fibromyalgia is made. The eighteen trigger points reflect areas through the spine and skeleton, which, over time, are repeatedly provoked into an expression of inflammation and pain. These are the same areas where tension with movement is usually noticed, as well as where 'usual and customary' structural misalignment patterns are found in the majority of humans. We are all subject to the same general, everyday, physical stresses of walking upright, sitting in weird positions, stretching into even more weird positions, sleeping crooked, bouncing around in various modes of transportation, walking on concrete – those kind of every day structural-impact activities.

The structural misalignment patterns represented by those eighteen points are similar to those found in our chiropractic patients with Chronic Sacroiliac Syndrome. Further, the structural and metabolic problems presented by Chronic Sacroiliac Syndrome patients often sounded similar to those presented by our already-diagnosed fibromyalgia patients.

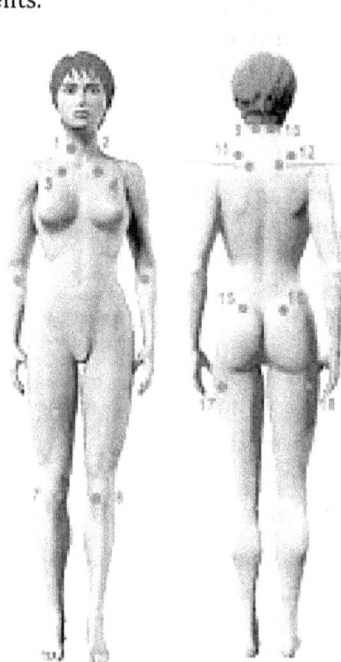

18 Myofascial Trigger Points

By the time eleven or more trigger points are involved, multiple body regions with this patient have become misaligned and dysfunctional, one with another (i.e.: low back accompanied by headaches and sinus or TMJ problems, not to mention knee and/or feet problems). This grouping of symptoms is an indication that the structural misalignment patterns have been accumulating for a long period of time and may have provoked the entire body structure, including its cranial and abdominal contents, to go awry... sometimes decidedly awry. If left untreated, the pattern can create a twist within the structure, set-off all kinds of nerve chaos causing nerve signals to mis-fire all over the body! By the time this full-body misconfiguration happens, multiple structural systems, such as the nervous systems and hormonal systems and liver systems and gastrointestinal systems, cannot work properly. People with these levels of problems are in PAIN! It's called *fibromyalgia*... but is it 'True' or 'Faux?'

In Separating 'True' From 'Faux'

Being able to diagnose the fibromyalgia condition doesn't necessarily mean the condition is a 'disease.' It is not unusual to hear many of the problems that are concerns of fibromyalgia patients being expressed by chronic sacroiliac syndrome patients: things such as a small bowel disturbance, sleeplessness, mid back pain, plantar fasciitis, acid reflux, anxiety, chronic headache, frequent sinus congestion, chest pain, knee pain, generalized body aches, low back pain, fatigue, etc. So many problems are overlapping, but all have to do with a nervous system disturbance. When the nervous system is disturbed, ALL of the body's systems are vulnerable to disruption.

What happens next can be likened to a domino effect: misalignment patterns around the human skeleton lead to a disturbed nervous system which, when left untreated, leads to circulatory chaos and slowly-increasing/expanding organ dysfunction leading to possible production of misalignment patterns. Added to that mix are the influences of eating, sleeping and behavioral habits of each individual. With this information, it is easy to determine the sources of so many varied problems. We have learned we need to address them all, starting with the basics.

- **Correct the structure (removing or lowering the neural chaos).**
- **Feed the cells (therapeutic levels of the basic seven nutrients).**

- **Remove the havoc makers (stop the everyday 'dosing' of foods or environments that create inflammatory conditions).**

Existence of active trigger points tells us that multiple structural regions of that body are involved. The points of pain tell us which regions of the body are involved. The regions involved tell us which nerves are involved, and the nerves involved tells us (Chiropractic Physicians) where and how to make an adjustment. **Correction of structural misalignments improves structural integrity, corrects neurological dysfunction, and allows symptoms to stop agitating, to fade away so parts can heal, allowing body regions to begin working together and functioning as a 'whole' again.** Structural integrity allows body regions to work as closely as possible to their 'normal' functions. The whole body begins to effectively function *together*. Almost too simple a concept, isn't it?

This book is not meant to disparage or simplify any pain or types of pain patterns felt by any person. Nor is it meant to place any doubt on the diagnostic procedures used by traditional western medicine, nor any of their research. Chiropractic physicians use most of the same diagnostic tools as well. You will learn how chiropractic research is different from - but *not* in opposition to - the physiology, neurology and circulatory descriptions evolving from medical research. Chiropractic analysis and structural medicine adds an additional layer to the diagnostic insight: the layer of neurological functioning with its structural empowerment. The intent is to define pain patterns in a way not yet widely discussed. What happens with the human structure when using structural and nutritional correction of the body's actions as part of the regular treatment plan is the element missing from the national conversations on fibromyalgia. Hopefully the definitions and descriptions provided in this book will be seen as another important layer to the conversation.

The Ol' Country Doc

You see, no one told the 'Little Country Doc' in me that I couldn't get people out of pain – particularly the pain of fibromyalgia. My purpose in becoming a Chiropractic Physician had never been to focus on research or academic study. The year I became a doctor, I celebrated thirty years in nursing: two-thirds of that time dedicated to acute care nursing in emergency rooms, operating rooms and intensive care units of our western hospitals. The ol' nurse in me, newly combined with the new doctor in me, had a Mission of "getting people out of pain, and helping them to live healthy lives." So I set about to do it!

Frustrated by the predominant and ongoing use of narcotics by traditional western medicine as a prescription for chronic pain, I opened the Fibromyalgia Care Center of Oregon in 1998. At that point in history, Oregon was third in the nation for the highest usage of methadone. It was the same year the Oregon Task Force for Pain and Symptom Management was in charge of finding out why. After 10 meetings around our state – and a year's worth of testimony from fibromyalgia patients about the degree to which narcotics were NOT solving the problem – the Taskforce put forth a statement suggesting the same policies continue that had been used for the last 30 years: *"treat pain with narcotics to the point of addiction and then treat the addiction."*

As I had observed through my years as a nurse, using narcotics to treat unremitting pain was the norm rather than to refer their chronic pain populace to physicians *whose main skill and expertise was in getting people out of pain!* The skills and techniques and natural remedies that could (and still can) be applied to ease the plight of the people who testified at those meetings were being completely ignored. Structurally and nutritionally, there are *so many* ways to get people out of pain, never mind living healthy lives. As a chiropractic physician, I have an arsenal of many ways to temper and gently eliminate pain patterns. The continued drugging of America incensed me. I set about to show it could be done... without drugs.

Taking Care Of The Whole

My years as a bedside nurse left me with a strong awareness of the numerous 'small' problems people tend to ignore, even as they cascade into the disordered conditions that develop into full-blown disease. Those 'small problems' are often the same concerns that prevent a person from resting, that agitate and grow into larger problems. Aches, pains and dysfunction will quietly accumulate over the course of days and weeks and years because of the thinking that *"my aches and pains and dysfunctions are not important enough to address"* or *"It's not so bad that I can't manage it."* Over and over again, I've witnessed the irritations of 'small' problems' sabotage the bigger picture of a person's health. Having to 'deal' with the little problems saps a person from being able to deal with the big ones when they come along. Sapping of your reserves actually makes you more vulnerable to bigger collapses. For example, when constipation or vitamin D deficiencies are not addressed and corrected, attempts to control infection or cancer prevention cannot be effective. How many people do you know have ongoing sinusitis or cellulites or bursitis or 'name-a-chronic-issue?' How many people do you know have on-going back or extremity pain? And how many also have accompanying complaints of adverse health in one way or another?

When an elbow joint isn't working properly, the knee joint can begin to dysfunction, causing a torque in the pelvis, adversely twisting the spine and all of its nerve trunks, ultimately involving the whole body and its functions – all the result of ignoring aches and pains along the way.

A Different Model

Looking beyond the traditional medical model of addressing the patient's symptoms and physiologic state of problematic disease, here at the Fibromyalgia Care Center of Oregon, we approach the body as a 'whole,' looking for the *cause* of symptoms and what provokes a physiologic state of disease. We find and correct structural misalignments. We feed the nutritionally missing components. We explore for environmental toxins and eliminate them. In ways beyond our wildest expectations, our multi-layered whole-body approach that had been consistently rectifying the structural and nutritional problems of Chronic Sacroiliac Syndrome also quieted fibromyalgia! All phases of it! People got back into their lives! And without DRUGS!

The *Healthy* Human Body

Years of repeated studies have found that when the human body is 1) kept structurally intact (thus *biomechanically, neurologically* and *physiologically* intact), 2) provided with adequate amounts of basic nutritional fuel, and 3) kept away from things that cause dysfunction, not only will the body survive, it will THRIVE! Ignore any one (or all) of these three components over the course of a lifetime and, though your body may withstand the stressors for a while, in due course, it will become *very* cranky with you. As you age and mature, it will have a greater and greater difficulty defending itself from disease and structural degeneration. Additionally, the body's rate and degree of aging will increase exponentially.

Could the structural dys-integrity we speak of be the basis of our current Baby Boomer's prevalence toward lifestyle diseases involving the lungs, heart or other abdominal organs? You may be surprised to hear that: **structural dysfunction is in fact known to be as much of a contributor to the development of lifestyle-related diseases as food intake and exercise habits.**

Health Of The Boomers

Early in the 1960s, as the boomers entered their teenage years, the American Medical Association (AMA) began playing a 'dirty trick' on the American people. They began a marketing campaign to discredit the chiropractic profession. The objective was to "contain and eliminate chiropractic."

Designed as a whisper campaign, spreading doubt about chiropractic medicine was the stratagem the AMA used to create fear about chiropractors. All doctors working with the whole body know that (barring trauma) structural pain is often the last to come and the first to go. During those decades, when chiropractors advised people to get adjusted periodically in order to maintain structural integrity, the medical (allopathic) community countered with, "if there's no pain how can there be a problem?" These two opposing philosophies created a generation of Americans to go on unnecessarily living with pain as well as numerous unresolved physical issues.

11

Creating doubt can be a powerful controller. For general, every-day aches and pains of their kids, parents of the boomers were taught: "just give them an aspirin, they'll be fine." That approach added the belief or understanding that pharmaceutical medicines could be used anytime. The AMA's adroit marketing campaign suc-ceeded in teaching the Boomers to 1) ignore structural problems and 2) pharmaceutically medicate – and hide – these same prob-lems, allowing another generation to believe that no pain meant no problem. Boomers failed to learn that those problems were signs of an increasingly malfunctioning body.

During those years, medical practice became defined as address-ing *symptoms only*, rather than by addressing the *actual causes of abnormal body function.* Medical treatment was no longer defined as finding and eliminating *the root cause of the problem*, just by *elimi-nating the symptom.* There are several arguments against this approach. From a chiropractic viewpoint, when a structural prob-lem is subdued through the use of a medication, and not structurally corrected, the adjacent body region (either above or below – which-ever is most vulnerable) is weakened and will begin to develop problems, pain or pathology. This is one of the ways pain and dis-ease slowly spread through the body.

The Marketing Of Health

The Boomers were also quietly taught to believe that taking nutri-tional supplements was unnecessary. *"You get all you need from your food"* was a popular saying. At that point in our national his-tory, the Recommended Daily Allowance (RDA) of nutritional levels was a large part of what national health education sources taught as being appropriate.

"Don't worry about any problem, your doctor has a pill for it!" was another implied message marketed to Boomers during the '60s and '70s. During that era, the pharmaceutical industry was expanding further and further into everyday life, while research about foods and/or human nutritional needs and benefits had come to a stand-still. Even in *today's* 2013 medical schools, medical doctors, nursing students AND pharmaceutical students still have only minimal to no exposure to the knowledge about the basic *nutritional* needs of the human body.

Through the '70s and '80s and '90s, many Americans continued to accept and believe the message that "nutritional supplementation is unnecessary." At the same time, an ever-increasing American interest in competitive sports had many of the Boomer generation attempting to live life to the fullest... with some going, too frequently and disastrously, beyond the limits of their body. Our stoic American men tended to ignore any structural injury short of a fracture. Full living ranged between too little activity and too much activity, often combined with minimal to no nutritional support. This is simply the type of lifestyle many Americans followed during those decades. As it turns out, ignoring structural and nutritional deficiencies actually increases the vulnerability of the human body in its ability to both develop disease and withstand disease.

Two Microscopes Looking at the Same Body

In the last several years, a good amount of the research studies conducted by the AMA have focused on the neurological components of fibromyalgia and its nerve and circulatory physiology. Though fascinating and excellent research, those medical discoveries reflect what the chiropractic profession has known for many years about the neurological expression of the human body. Since its inception, chiropractic medicine has recognized the effects from the ongoing presence of inflammation with its structural compromise as a natural consequence of pathological disease processes. As structural neurologists, chiropractors are all about improving the nervous system and its functions.

Fibromyalgia research is one area that demonstrates the difference in focus between the two health disciplines: traditional western medical research compared with chiropractic research. Both have strong relevance, yet each focuses on a different aspect of the same problem.

Once a condition has been established as a disease, medical research will focus on the specific diseased area of the body (such as conducting a focused study on the liver, kidney or heart) in an effort to pinpoint a singular organ dysfunction causing the symptoms. They will develop a strategy – usually a surgical procedure or pharmaceutical prescription drug – to calm the symptoms. Sometimes the solution is to remove a certain body part or organ.

13

On the other hand, chiropractic research focuses on the entire system, seeing it as a 'whole,' where "the whole is greater than the sum of its parts." Chiropractors, knowing our nerves follow all the major bony paths, survey the entire body structure and its nerve function, as well as take into account a person's lifestyle. The cause of symptom expression is found through a comprehensive health history, examination, postural assessment, neurological evaluation, palpation, imaging, etc. Then chiropractors can effectively treat and correct the specific areas that require attention. Correcting nerve function through chiropractic adjustments and manipulation techniques replaces nerve chaos with nerve tranquility and chemical balance in the body. This removes the root cause of the problem and promotes improvement to the power supply of the body to organs and other parts. More often than not, this approach and application eliminates symptoms, puts a smile on *Jane Doe's* face and lets her walk away, restored back toward health.

Chiropractic research focuses on 1) what the body doesn't have or isn't getting enough of (deficiency), 2) what impedes the body's natural functions (toxicity, and/or nerve interference), and 3) the structural/nerve condition that causes the body to develop a particular condition or disease. Doctors of Chiropractic treat the symptom back to its root cause, back to the precise area of the body that has dysfunction. For example, if the kidney presents with disease, chiropractors evaluate the nerve function at the vertebral level that supplies power to the kidney. Research shows that when the power source (the particular nerve) isn't working, the associated organ will begin to sputter, dysfunction or degenerate, and possibly fail. The body's cellular chemistry is distorted. Lab values will change and a disease can be diagnosed.

Yes, the problem could certainly be an esoteric pesticide or bacterium introduced to the body, but that rationale and approach merely addresses the element of toxicity. It neglects to recognize the human body as the self-healing and self-regulating organism that it can be when it is structurally intact. What allowed that pesticide or bacterium to take hold? Why did that body let it in? When you hear a stampede, *think horses not zebras*. Meaning, address and correct the most possible and obvious probabilities *first* rather than chase after an unusual or rare condition that *might* occur. For example, the nerves that serve the immune system are located in the mid-back; if

14

your back is twisted, causing them to lose nerve power, the immune function is compromised. Do you think that could be why the bacterium could initially take hold and you suddenly developed pneumonia? The nerves in the neck feed all the parts of the head and face; if those nerves are lacking power, could that be a cause of hearing deficiency and/or your migraine headaches? Or could it be part of what caused you to come down with your most recent cold or flu? If you unplugged the cord of your coffee maker, would it still make coffee? In the same way, the body's power (nerve) supply couldn't perform its normal functions without a connection to its source: the nervous system.

Chiropractors remove potentially toxic elements, replenish deficiencies, restore nerve function, and get out of the way to allow the body to do what it does best: heal itself from the inside out, naturally.

Both approaches (allopathic and chiropractic) have a time and place for application. One treats disease when disease occurs, and the other promotes healthy body function, tempering the development of disease. One puts out the fire, the other restores the structure, preventing potential for another fire. Both are needed in our country. Both are necessary. During a crisis or trauma, there is no better medicine than the practice of allopathic physicians. However, with chronic structural problems, either structural or metabolic, allopathic medicine may not be the best place to start your health care. After fifty-two years of service in both health care arenas, my experience has taught me that reaching for structural integrity is the best place to start before any other type of treatment. When you have 'a hitch in your get-along,' take care of the "hitch" and see how your "get along" improves.

The Evolution Of Insight

The work, research and findings expressed in this book are the result of discoveries made during my 20+ years of practice as a chiropractic physician... yes, preceded by all as those years of bedside and acute care nursing. During my years as a chiropractor, it has been an honor to base my work on the structural and physiological findings of Dr. Major Bertram DeJarnette, and the Sacral Occipital body patterns discovered through his research.

Considered a genius of his era, Dr. DeJarnette was licensed both as a Doctor of Osteopathy and a Doctor of Chiropractic. Avidly interested in research, he was fastidiously disciplined with documenting his clinical observations and procedures. Working closely with Dr. George Goodheart and other brilliant minds of that era, Dr. DeJarnette added numerous valuable chiropractic *and* medical understandings, some still in use in clinical practice today. Our understanding of the anatomy of spinal nerves came from his research (see *Spinal Nerve Map*).

Dr. DeJarnette's 73 years of focused research left us with a treasure trove of understanding about the human skeleton, its neurology and physiology. Not only did his work show how the skeleton and its surrounding structures fit together, but also how they influence one another, working together as a whole, each part in turn requiring the support of the body part above and/or below. Dr. DeJarnette's extensive collection of data portrays structural patterns that demonstrate how our 206 +/- bones, 600 some odd muscles, all the connective tissue and fascia, together with about a billion of our finest nerves and blood vessels, all manage to work synergistically!

Dr. DeJarnette's insights into the structural system, collectively known as the Sacral Occipital Technique (SOT), provide a clear understanding of the **connection between structural dysfunctions and the development of disease.** It's an excellent basis for understanding how un-corrected layers of dysfunction allow structural stress to accumulate, increase the *cellular* stress and lead to organ compromise. Today, more and more research demonstrates the link between metabolic diseases and those layers of uncorrected structural dysfunction. Structural dysfunction compromises nerve action, nerve flow, and nerve facilitation, thus slowly destroying health. (www.sorsi.com, www.sotousa.com)

As a chiropractor, using Sacral Occipital Technique (SOT), with both its diagnostic and treatment potentials, I began to recognize the structural patterns fostered by the common diseases in our society. Using the parameters and testing of SOT, it was quickly obvious how skeletal dysfunction allows structural stress to accumulate, increasing *cellular* stress, leading to the types of organ compromise we call diabetes or colitis or psoriatic arthritis or heart

16

valve displacement or acid reflux or plantar fasciitis or (fill in the blank with the name of *your* disease). SOT taught me to recognize how structural integrity – or the lack thereof - influences health and/or the development of organ compromise. With this as a basis for understanding, coupled with the fact that Americans get so little chiropractic care, it is easy to recognize why and how people have become such a diseased and arthritic populace.

In The Common Patterns

Of the many contributions Dr. DeJarnette brought to our understanding of the human body, the one I appreciate most is the structural condition discussed throughout this book. The contribution is the recognition that (barring trauma) humans tend to walk and drive around in a similar universe, developing similar biomechanical patterns. Each of us has a unique version according to how we live our lives. Our biomechanical patterns influence our structural body, and when our patterns become offset, they create structural misalignments and neurologic weaknesses in the body. While not normal – nor predictable – dysfunctional *patterns* are common across our population. When they last longer than six months, they're considered *chronic*. When grouped together as a pattern, the weaknesses and misalignments are known as a *syndrome*. When a group of signs and symptoms stem from and surrounds the pelvis, it is considered to be a *sacroiliac joint dysfunction*, making the chronic sacroiliac syndrome (CSS) the most common misalignment pattern known.

The Chronic Sacroiliac Syndrome, Also Known As 'Faux' Fibromyalgia

Dr. DeJarnette helped us to recognize the importance of the progression of slow, minute, *gradual* changes that occur or cascade through the human skeletal structure in response to an individual's daily lifestyle and environment. Everyone is subject to similar forces in our universe such as gravity, vibrational compression (compression from riding in a vehicle, bumps, bangs and/or falls), plus the continual compression accumulated from walking on hard surfaces. During the cumulative buildup of these forces, a generic pattern of structural dysfunction can often develop. A person's lifestyle largely determines how the cascade progresses, in which *pattern* the cascade occurs, and the *degree* of dysfunction the cascade causes.

While there are common triggering forces that cause similar patterns of distortion, each person's response is unique. Daily lifestyle (occupation, nutritional diet, exercise, and other habits), combined with the emotional, traumatic, and environmental factors unique to each person's universe collectively contribute to how a person responds to their internal and external changes. Changing to internal and external environments is known as adaptation. A person's ability or inability to adapt impacts and influences their skeletal structure and genetic expression. **Structure determines function; function determines structure.**

Snugly Fit Together!

Dr. Gunther von Hagen's presentation of Body Worlds, Inc. (www.bodyworlds.com), developed a unique method for removing connective tissues and fat from (donated) cadavers. For the first time ever, this incredible technique called *Plastination* allows us to observe the inside of the human body. In Dr. von Hagen's *Bodyworks* exhibits, models of the human body are positioned in an activity of life such as the stance used when shooting a bow and arrow, held in a specific position suspended from motion, as though they were caught in a freeze-frame snapshot: feet shoulder width apart, body perpendicular to the shooting line and target, one shoulder pointing toward the target, one hand pulling back the bowstring, the other holding the bow, with fingers lightly holding the arrow on the string "split finger" style. One can visualize the dynamics of the body's inner parts, its co-dependent muscles and bones synergistically at work, poised for action. *Bodyworks* is a stunning display of the utterly beautiful human body's intricate functions with every-day tasks.

Coaxial Cable Construction

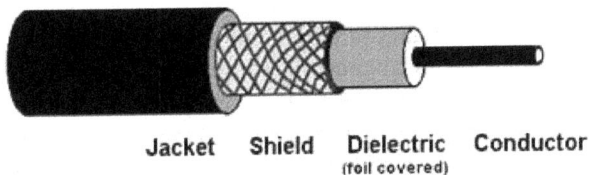

Jacket   Shield   Dielectric   Conductor
(foil covered)

Conceptualize the similarities between the body and a coaxial cable. Our skin holds our inner parts tightly together like a coaxial cable's outer plastic sheath; muscles beneath the skin act like a woven copper shield beneath the plastic sheath, bones like an inner dielectric insulator, and nerves like the copper core – with little to no space between each part. Every part has a position and its dimensions have grown to exactly the right size for what it needs to do and for the space in which it has to live amongst the community of all the other body parts. It is exactly the right size, in exactly the right place, and has to be in order to do exactly what it needs to do when it is called to do it. All of our body's mechanisms and parts fit just as snugly together, like an organized pattern.

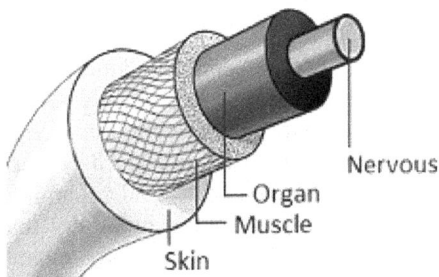

Nervous
Organ
Muscle
Skin

Take away the skin to visualize all our parts, blood vessels and nerves (the pipes and wires), with all their muscles, tendons and fascial fibers (the pulleys and cords), and all other innervating nerves (the power supply) fitting appropriately together and you'll see there is a place for everything and everything has a place. Truly, no extra space exists for anything other than being in the right place at the right time. There's no space to move out of order without having an effect on another part. Each part is supposed to be in its own place.

Applying this spatial fact to understanding how a bony misalignment or a *group* of misalignments can create problems in other areas of the body, such as with a kneecap shifting a quarter inch to the left. Muscles attached to bones, and nerves intertwine between muscles and organs, in a similar manner to the way the parts of a coaxial cable fit together. Nerves cannot withstand pressure or kinking, just as cables cannot take sharp bends, as the shield would kink, causing losses in the cable. In like manner, if a nerve is pinched or kinked, it has a loss of function. Look at a cadaver after Plastination; you can see a misalignment wouldn't need to be very big to cause a disruption. The body is not designed with enough room for misalignments, not to mention *patterns* of them! All those pipes and wires and pulleys and fibers don't like to be stretched or buckled... it makes them work funny... or not at all.

Ignoring cause?

Knowing misalignments influence health so drastically, how can the effects of accumulated compactions of various joints throughout the skeletal structure be ignored? Structural misalignments can be seen in nearly every x-ray performed.

These types of pain patterns aren't the kind of thing that can be corrected by a pill. Narcotics don't fully relieve pain; they allow the pain to be tolerated to a greater degree but don't fully relieve it. Pills may pacify the pain patterns, but only until the accumulation of misalignment patterns with their residual inflammatory chemical debris become so chronic (and further inflamed) that the pills are no longer effective; more and more pills are needed in order to reach the same level of effectiveness. That pain pattern could not, at any point or in any way, be *corrected* through the use of any pill.

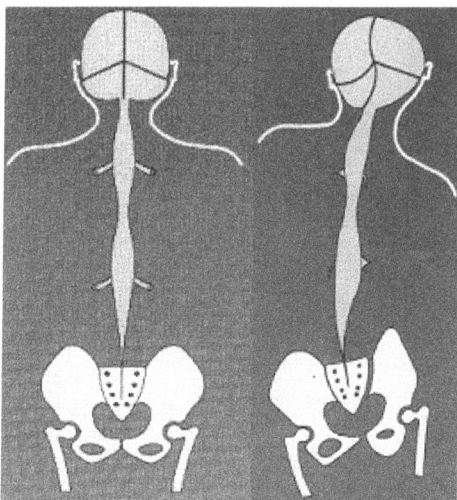

Normal Posture (left) verses Abnormal Posture (right).

Being so focused into disease and with their many chemical and surgical treatments, medical doctors rarely consider the structural connection to the onset of pain. **The element ignored**, yet to be embraced by medical practitioners, **is the degree of restoration to the healthy function of biochemistry and natural physiology that follows correction of the structure.** Chiropractors watch the reduction of pain and inflammation through structural correction every day. Pain patterns are reduced and often eliminated entirely.

Which is why I decided to 1) write this book, and 2) write it directly to the people needing this important information: YOU, the people. It is written to you, who want to be well, who want to be out of pain; to you, who want to live your life with joy and delight and sparkle; to you, who want to dance; to you, who want to live your life *without addiction* to pharmaceutical drugs; to you, who want to live in health!

2

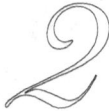

Dale de Madison

"IF you can't explain it simply, you don't understand it well
enough."
~ *Albert Einstein*

Misalignments & Structural Distortion

Using his wife as a prop (while attempting to appear as though he
wasn't using his wife as a prop), Dale walked into my office leaning
to the left at such an angle I thought he might topple-over. With each
step, his right arm reached to make contact with anything stable. His
face was so pinched with the effort of holding himself upright the
whites of his eyes could barely be seen. Keeping his eyes open was
almost impossible due to the swirling of his brain; but to close them
increased his vulnerability to falling. To stay upright, he was forced
to carry his head to the left, almost to the level of his left shoulder.

He described his headaches as "migraines with auras" occurring
on the average of once to twice a month for the past forty years! His
headaches had actually been going on longer than the vertigo.

Of course he'd visited every type of medical doctor possible and
had every probe, scan and test available – all showing "*nothing of
significance.*" He'd been taking many medications, some for numer-

ous years, with the vertigo continuing unresolved. It never really became too much worse, but didn't get any better either.

His wife, already a patient in our office for over two years, had wanted him to come in to see me. From her own experience, she knew I could help him. But at first he didn't want to have anything to do with our approach. He had no confidence that chiropractic medicine would know anything about his problem that could make a difference in his situation. After all, he'd already "been to a dozen of the best neurologists around the state and they couldn't find anything." He had no understanding of the depth of a chiropractor's ability to help him, much less the capabilities of a skilled craniopath.

Turns out, Dale was a forester. At the age of fifty-nine when he walked into our office, he was closing on retirement and "just needed to make it another six months" to secure his pension. The episodes of the vertigo he battled were occurring "about once to twice a month" over the last *thirty years*! He had a loss of hearing and acknowledged a constant ringing in both ears. He also stated he occasionally experienced nausea with the vertigo, but "it never went any further" to cause vomiting.

I asked him, "How do you manage both your exaggerated lean to the left *and* the swirling in your brain?"

He told me, "I just walked carefully. Up until two months ago, it wasn't so bad that I couldn't get through it." However, with the recent escalation of his symptoms he was concerned he would not be able to 'make it until retirement.'

He couldn't remember any type of trauma or accident or fall occurring recently, but he did tell me about a fall at the age of fourteen where he "injured the middle of his back on the left side." He also acknowledged, that, as a forester, he often walked along sloping terrain. He explained a game he used to practice, of "keeping his left foot on the higher side" walking lopsided. This repeated game, over thirty-odd years caused him to lean left into a slope, fostered an accumulation of structural (skeletal) misalignments, setting the stage for a pattern of chronic distortion that cascaded throughout his entire spine and body. This pattern ultimately affected even his cranium, causing a curved distortion of his head, which appeared kidney shaped. It was one of the more profound cranial distortions I'd ever seen.

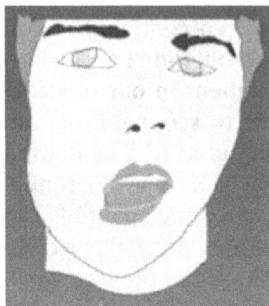

Cranial Distortion

Cranial Distortion

When looking at him face to face, Dale's head literally appeared concave. It looked like a kidney, with his left eye being the center or concave side of the kidney. The inner aspect of his left eye was scrunched towards his nose with his nose physically pulling to the left. His left cheek was pulled back into his face and toward his nose. The right side of his mouth was lower than the left side and the wrinkles on the left were deeply ingrained. His head leaned so far to the left his neck was curved into a side-ways C-shape.

More interesting to me, was when I pointed this out to him, Dale looked at me and very honestly said: "Hmm, I never noticed that."

His wife agreed with Dale. While she always noticed him scrunching his left eye, she hadn't realized how severe the scrunching had become. Once it was pointed out to her, she was astonished at how distorted his face and cranium appeared. I don't often see – or treat – this degree of cranial distortion.

With the antagonistic attitude prevailing in our country regarding any treatment other than traditional western medicine, many people are diverted away from the structural arena before they ever even walk into our office. Too many people are unaware that there are doctors highly skilled in the assessment, diagnosis and correction of the cranium. We are called Craniopaths and have been known to change a person's life – for the positive – using only our hands as tools.

All The Way To The Head?

The human body is a malleable unit. It can move and shift, and can literally and structurally adapt to its environment. Because the body is constructed with two halves (discussed more in the next chapters), skeletal misalignments can cause one half to 'droop.' When your chiropractor tells you that you have 'a short leg,' it is not meant to imply you have a leg that is (anatomically) shorter. Instead, it means you have developed skeletal changes at your pelvis causing one leg to appear shorter than the other. One side of your pelvis is drooping and the other pulling up.

As a 'short leg' disparity continues to develop – it's an *extremely* slow on-going process, nano-millimeter by nano-millimeter, happening sometimes over years, maybe decades. Yet as it develops, joints and other body parts will often begin dysfunctioning, as one side pushes up along the spine and ribs and the other side sags or droops away from the spine and ribs. This distortion between the two halves of the body creates a tractioning and/or crowding, a 'pushing-together' and/or 'pulling-apart' type of stress at the cellular levels of the involved body parts. The surrounding pipes, wires and paths (nerves, blood vessels and lymph channels) resonate that sense of *crowding* and *stretching*, no matter what system is being affected. Though a small distortion, it can change how muscles or body parts function, individually or as a group. More and more professionals are beginning to understand how this progressive structural distortion (with its resulting cascade of stress on connective tissue, muscles and organs) can set up the basic changes from which many diseases stem.

Slight on-going shifts in structure alter how cells and body parts relate within themselves and to one another. The shifting of bony structures pulls supportive ligaments, igniting pain receptors and causing muscles and/or fascia to 'bunch up' and/or stretch thinly. When muscles and fascia are not at their normal length, adhesions form in the tissue and cause stiffness – particularly in people who tend to be more sedate than active. Like a ripple in water, structural dysfunction can slowly spread throughout all body regions, including your head.

The Effects of Cranial Distortion

The same slow compression and stress that causes gradual development of the "short leg" disparity often instigates cranial distortion. With approximately 22 bones and about 47 joints, your skull can misalign just as readily as anything south. In the skull, however, misalignments affect the positioning of the brain. And that may change nerve expression and/or response to your environment, not to mention your individualized physical, mental, emotional, structural, and behavioral propensity.

Changes in the structural integrity of the cranium or skull, called Cranial Distortion, are the end result of multiple adaptations and structural shifts. Almost everyone who lives in gravity or rides in vehicles or walks on concrete, for any length of time, develops some degree of diagnosable cranial distortion.

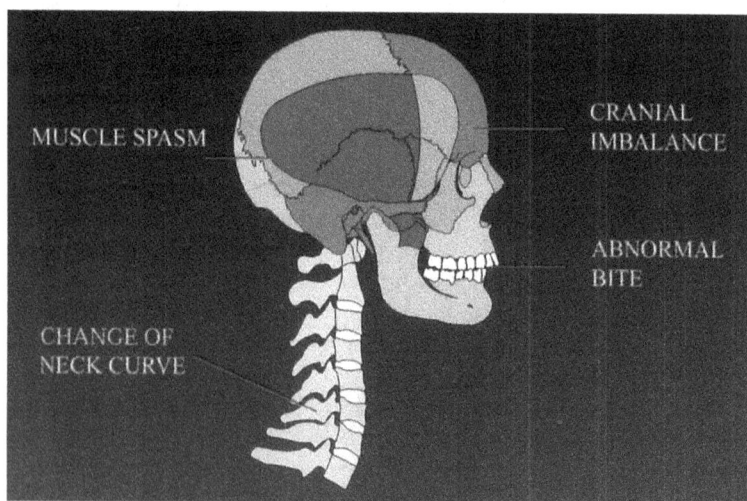

Notice the change in the jaw and the straightening of the cervical (neck) curve.

Certainly anyone who experiences global or regional headaches, sinus difficulties, earaches, TMJ problems, vertigo, Mennier's Disease (especially if increased with flying), snoring, sleep apnea or any variety of mood disorders likely has a degree of cranial distortion.

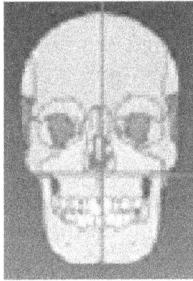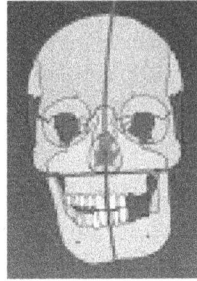

Normal	*Distorted*

Think about it for a minute: the twelve cranial nerves that provide power and sensation to your face and power for the automatic rhythms of your body (seeing, hearing, breathing, sleeping, digesting, hormonal production, thinking, etc.) live and work in your skull. If your head can twist and torque a bit, wouldn't that set up some problems for the two halves of the brain to communicate? Could that disparity be contributing to the prevalence of *bipolar disorder*?

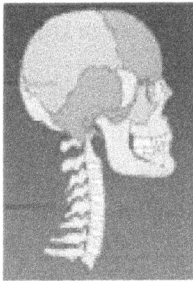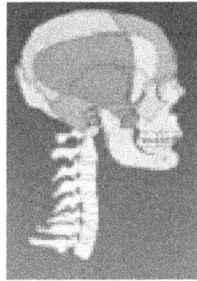

Normal	*Distorted*

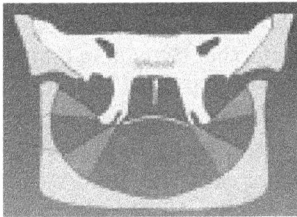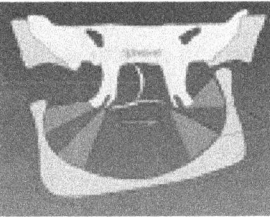

Normal	*Distorted*

Question: What happens to your personal productivity when you're crowded or twisted around in your living space? It becomes bogged-down, right? You stop getting so much done, don't you? I don't function very well in those conditions either. Cranial distortion crowds cranial nerves in much the same way, changing their nerve output.

That crowding pulls on the nerves and dura (the balloon-like lining surrounding the brain), in turn adding to the complexity of the cranial distortion. This Dural Torque can be responsible for a variety of pain and problems. Migraine headaches, of numerous varieties, are the result of this Dural Torque. The result can be dysfunction of any or all of the brain organs (such as the centers of your brain that control emotion, speech, vision, hearing, regulation of breathing, circulation and hormone production) and ventricles (your gyroscopes). Could this distortion be why you have frequent headaches? Or why you are sleeping so poorly? Anyone who needs a C-pap machine to sleep has some degree of cranial distortion present, affecting his or her cranial nerve power output. Could misalignment of cranial bones – and the often-accompanying Dural Torque – be the spark for epileptic seizures or other types of brain spasm?

Everyday Evolvement Of Cranial Distortion

Anyone who experiences low back pain or pain down the back of their legs or in their pelvis or at their mid-back or across their shoulders will also commonly develop some degree of cranial distortion. When one end of the spine is stressed, over time the other end will reflect that stress. What affects the spine will ultimately affect the cranium. Fortunately, most all of the time, it is correctable!

When cranial distortion is not addressed along with the rest of the body during chiropractic adjustments, that remaining cranial distortion can, over time, pull the lower body back into its previous misalignment pattern. Maybe not quite to the same degree, but it will certainly influence the body back into the basic pattern it had developed through the years. Cranial correction and stability does appear to be one of the factors contributing to the ability of the rest of the skeleton to maintain its alignment.

Structural misalignment patterns are a fact of everyday life for every person. And, just as every part of the body must work together to make the whole body function properly, some misalignment patterns can keep the body in dysfunction if not corrected in a timely manner. In other words, when you treat one problem in the body, you really want to address all of the problems, as a residual problem can perpetuate or stimulate another.

Misalignment patterns compromise and interrupt nerve flow. They twist, torque, buckle and/or traction nerves. A nerve being stressed in this way affects the production of neurotransmitters, which affects whole regions of the nervous system. When nerve flow is compromised, environmental, nutritional and/or microbial stressors are able to overwhelm the metabolic system, setting the stage for the development of any number of diseases in the human system. The cranium carries the majority of the stimulus for the body's nervous systems. Since it houses 80% of your nerve output, wouldn't it be important to adjust the cranial distortion too?

What Causes Misalignments?

While there is similarity to the variety of patterns that evolve from living in our shared universe, each body is unique with its own unique set of misalignment patterns. The type of misalignments that develop depends on a variety of lifestyle factors: occupation, eating habits, exercise habits, etc. Are you the person throwing your body around the universe, or very carefully stepping off each curb? Do you eat fresh fruits and veggies on a daily basis or hit the fast food drive-through along your way? Have you been abused either psychologically or physically? Are you including yourself into the practice of family health care? Or do you ignore yourself, taking care of yourself last, if at all?

Cranial Distortion And Traumatic Brain Injury

All of those factors, and dozens of others, influence the type of misalignment patterns that occur in any particular structure. Truth be told, nobody goes without developing and/or experiencing some type of misalignment pattern on a daily basis.

The skull is as vulnerable to misalignment as any other part of the body, perhaps even more. ANY traumatic hit or blow will distort the skull, changing nerve output. ALL traumatic brain injuries involve the dura and the cranial plates. Every concussion needs cranial care and correction. Chiropractic care needs to be made available to any child hit on a sport's field. So much talent is wasted and damage allowed by avoiding this level of structural correction. Post Traumatic Stress Disorder (PTSD) is often tempered with correction of cranial distortion. Chiropractic service should be routinely available to US soldiers as soon as any trauma occurs. In 2002, Congress mandated access to chiropractic care for all of our enlisted and wounded military personnel. Yet in 2014, most all of our veterans are still waiting for this level of sophisticated care.

Other Areas Where Improvement Is Seen After Cranial Correction

We've seen manic/depressive cycles slow and steady when the cranium is corrected, allowing the brain to sit squarely within its space. By sitting squarely, the bridge of the brain (the corpus callosum) can 'level,' allowing clearer and more consistent communication between both hemispheres of the brain. Could this improve the condition of schizophrenia? Just correcting the pain components of a brain trauma can set a person back on their road to life. This is precisely the reason chiropractic care, with craniopathy, needs to be a part of every psychiatric or psychological treatment plan. Until you correct cranial distortion, how do you know how much is physical dysfunction disrupting nerve communication and thought processing, verses how much is actually mental dysfunctioning? Put the cart before the horse.

Dale

By the way, remember Dale? It only took eight months to get his face and head looking normal – not to mention getting his head upright onto his neck, his nose straight, and to the point where he could walk upright with no left lean, no headaches and no vertigo. All with no surgery and no drugs! Using the magnificence of the doctor's hands as skillful tools. He still hasn't grasped the degree of the problem he had when we started the correction. But he is happily retired, walking upright – with a non-swirling head – and that works for me, and more importantly for him.

3

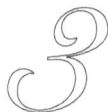

Acquired Fibromyalgia: 'Faux' Fibro

Becoming Known As 'Faux' Fibro

When Tammy first appeared in our office she was only 33, yet she looked 60. With the diagnosis of fibromyalgia four years prior, she began feeling life was hopeless. She thought she would forever have pain in her body. She sat slumped in her chair, with her first comments to me, "I have no energy. I hurt all the time. I feel like my head is going to explode."

Stories such as her collection of symptoms have become commonplace here at the Fibromyalgia Care Center of Oregon. They make my heart ache.

Tammy's particular story included a history of daily headaches radiating from the base of her head, over the top of her scalp, to the crest of her nose. As she sat with me on her first visit to my office, she told me, "I've had my current headache for the past three days. It ranges from a 3 to a 9" on a 10-point pain scale (10 being the most severe). "I experience this types of episode on average of 1 to 3 times a month." Her neck hurt from the base of her skull down to her diaphragm and her shoulders ached constantly; both her hands became numb if she sat for any length of time over ten minutes.

"And, oh, by the way," she added, "I've had a chronic sinus infection since the age of twelve." The pain between her shoulder blades was constant, described as an "8" on the 10-point pain scale. Her low back, she said, "is less painful than my neck" but she still had pain at both hips as well as at the outside and inside of both knees. "My joints ache constantly." And she added, "more often than not, the arches of my feet hurt so badly I can't walk."

Every trigger point was tender. Sleep? The thought of awakening rested was something she no longer believed could happen. Exhaustion felt like a constant companion. "It's like a blanket of pain around my shoulders." A tall, slim lady, she sat in front of me leaning forward, with her head held halfway to her knees.

Trauma had been a factor several times in her life, having gone through a rollover motor vehicle accident in high school, as well as a nasty inline-skating tussle about six years ago and a fairly serious rear-end car collision about two years ago. Yet, with all of this, the only treatment for her condition was a pharmaceutical intake of Excedrin.

Her food intake included three mocha lattes a week, with an "occasional *NutraSweet*" every week, and three to four 16-ounce glasses of water per day. Her nutritional supplementation intake consisted of one capsule of Glucosamine-chondroitin, 1,000 mg of calcium in tablet form, a B6, a B12 and "alternating tablets of calcium, zinc and magnesium every other day." This history tells me she was making an effort at keeping her body clean and drug-free, while giving it at least some of what the current public knowledge understands about nutritional support. Not at all bad and certainly not wrong. Yet a long way from complete – never mind what is necessary and effective to promote healing and adequate metabolic support.

She also had a long history of bruising easily. "I've always got a bruise somewhere on me." Because of her ongoing sinus infection, she told me, "It is easy for me to breakdown into a cold." (Immune difficulties always indicate nutritional shortages; colds often indicate food sensitivities.) Her monthly menses, heralded by several days of "serious PMS," included clotting within her flow, one to three days of cramping and "not-at-all-fun" mood swings. This history tells us more about the *degree* of her nutritional deficiencies. Her fatigue, anxiety and sleeplessness spoke LOUDLY to other nutritional deficiencies, possibly compounded by food reactions such as allergies or sensitivities.

Nutritional deficiencies will always be reflected in cartilage health, meaning: nutritional deficiencies foster pain and the development of restriction with joint movement, which are precursors to degenerative joint disease, also known as arthritis. The timeliness of her pain patterns tells us of possible food interactions and sensitivities. Combine nutritional deficiencies with neurological compromise created by the accumulation of structural misalignment patterns, and the body is restricted in its ability to either calm down or focus on the tasks of living and thriving. Instead it is forced to focus on surviving, repairing and rebuilding.

Food sensitivities cause cellular histamine (inflammation) to be continually released in a body's cellular systems, fostering, through the prostaglandin secretion system, an on-going cellular-nerve expression of pain and anxiety.

Overall, her history tells us she has developed a metabolic, possibly toxic, component to her structural pattern that is continually perpetuating her condition. This explanation doesn't seem adequate to summarize the tragedy it has caused in her life, does it? Yet it encompasses the truth of how accumulated structural misalignments – especially when combined with nutritional deficiencies and/or food sensitivities – add up to chronic structural pain.

Cartilage is the dense, tough, normally resilient tissue covering both sides of every joint and making up the discs in the spine, at the temporal-mandibular joints and at the pelvis. Cartilage is composed of tall, vertical, columns of cells. As an non-vascular tissue, it doesn't actually have a blood supply flowing directly to it. Nor does it have a direct nerve supply. Consequently, cartilage is dependent on the diffusion of fluid containing oxygen and nutrients from surrounding tissue to maintain its needed state of hydration. The strength of a disc and its ability to resist degeneration is dependent on its state of hydration, meaning the amount of water stored within its cells. The pumping action is dependent on physical activity and occurs in the cellular fields from movements like walking and/or other physical exercise.

The degree to which your cartilage is saturated is called 'hydration.' Hydration means the amount of water stored within its cells. Hydration determines the cartilage cell's internal strength and ability to hold and sway to the position your spine and back is seeking. The degree of that saturation starts with your water intake, proceeds through digestion and circulation. Then, through osmosis, your fluids saturate the cartilage, determining the height (and strength) of those

cartilage pads between your vertebra, at your jaw and in your pelvis.

The action of osmosis is promoted through activities such as walking, running, jumping, dancing, laughing, talking, singing, etc. Consequently, osmosis and/or pumping-like actions are essential to provide lubrication and hydration to the cellular fields in each disc and every region of cartilage. This need for hydration makes walking such a necessary function for the maintenance of health – and structural ease, strength and integrity in the human body.

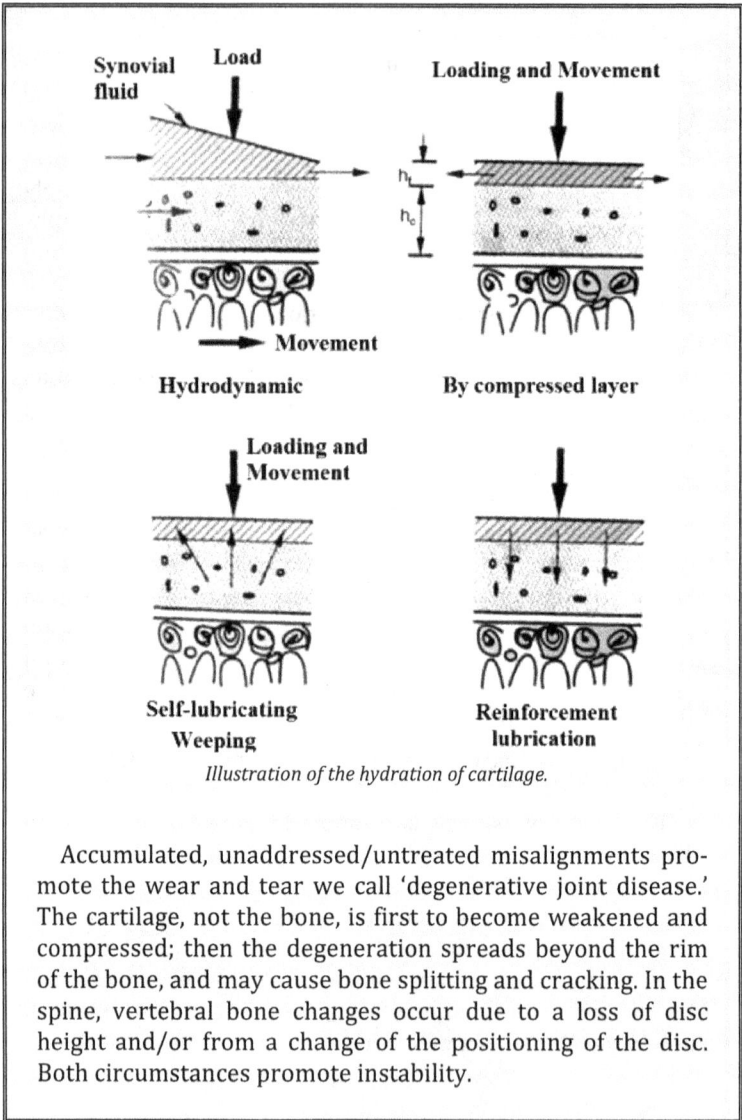

Illustration of the hydration of cartilage.

Accumulated, unaddressed/untreated misalignments promote the wear and tear we call 'degenerative joint disease.' The cartilage, not the bone, is first to become weakened and compressed; then the degeneration spreads beyond the rim of the bone, and may cause bone splitting and cracking. In the spine, vertebral bone changes occur due to a loss of disc height and/or from a change of the positioning of the disc. Both circumstances promote instability.

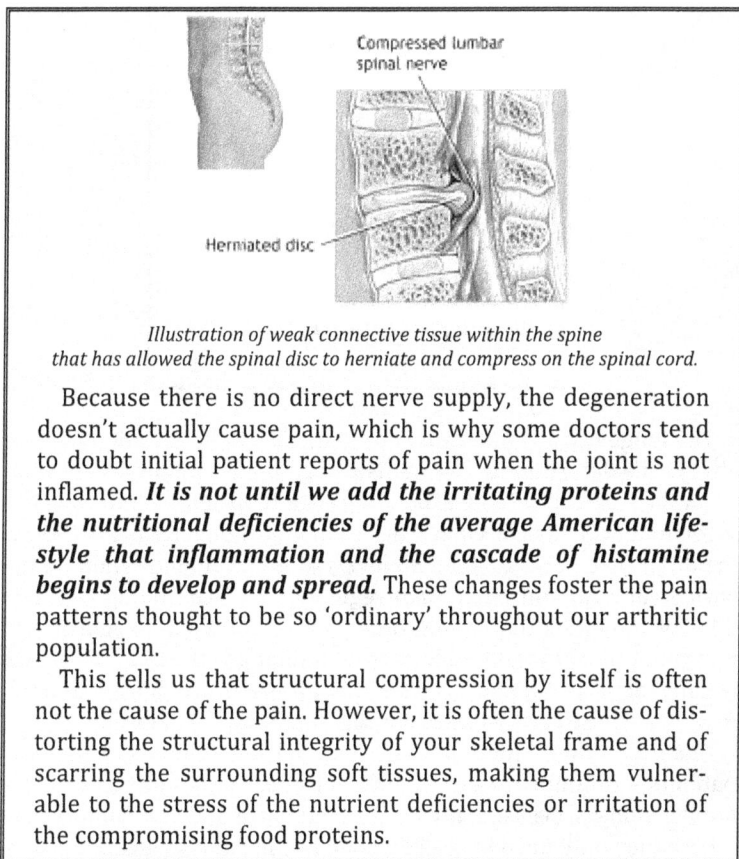

*Illustration of weak connective tissue within the spine
that has allowed the spinal disc to herniate and compress on the spinal cord.*

Because there is no direct nerve supply, the degeneration doesn't actually cause pain, which is why some doctors tend to doubt initial patient reports of pain when the joint is not inflamed. ***It is not until we add the irritating proteins and the nutritional deficiencies of the average American lifestyle that inflammation and the cascade of histamine begins to develop and spread.*** These changes foster the pain patterns thought to be so 'ordinary' throughout our arthritic population.

This tells us that structural compression by itself is often not the cause of the pain. However, it is often the cause of distorting the structural integrity of your skeletal frame and of scarring the surrounding soft tissues, making them vulnerable to the stress of the nutrient deficiencies or irritation of the compromising food proteins.

'True' Fibromyalgia or 'Faux' Fibromyalgia?

Our initial question with Tammy: is her condition a version of a 'True' Fibromyalgia or 'Faux' Fibromyalgia?

With five distinguished types of Fibromyalgia currently defined, the first step with each new patient is to identify the *type* of fibromyalgia being expressed: Acquired, Traumatic, Toxic, Metabolic, or Genetic.

---

5 Types of Fibromyalgia

- Aquired
- Traumatic
- Metabolic
- Toxic
- Genetic (?)

The longevity of a problem and/or its degree of chronicity are not always the determining factors. The degree of systemic (body-wide) inflammation can often be the difference between the two levels of involvement. I realize what I am saying still doesn't solidly define the difference between the two levels of involvement. When treated with structural and nutritional regimens, we are finding that over 80% of the cases that come to us - with a previous diagnosis and history of fibromyalgia - are back into their lives, out of pain, functioning at a far higher capacity than when we began working together. These are the cases we began calling Faux Fibros.

The other 25% – the ones we began to call the True Fibromyalgia patients – do improve but at a slower rate, some taking as long as twelve months, occasionally more, to stabilize and plateau to a point where they only need to see someone like me about once a month to once a quarter in order for their bodies to stay quiet, calmly out of pain and serving them in the manner of a 'normal' body.

Finding Out

Tammy went through an extensive examination including chiropractic, orthopedic, and neurologic testing that showed what she already knew: over time her range of motion had become compromised, resulting in positive findings on numerous chiropractic, orthopedic and neuromusculoskeletal tests. All eighteen of her Fibromyalgia Trigger Points were sensitive the day of her initial exam, but not all to the point of being labeled as 'active' trigger points.

That doesn't mean she wasn't in some serious pain; it simply says *the day of her initial exam* the trigger points didn't fit the 'active' criteria.

Acquired Fibromyalgia & Chronic Sacroiliac Syndrome Myofascial Trigger Points

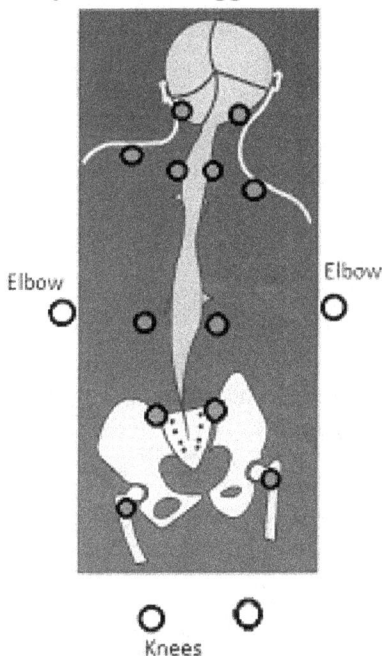

Elbow   Elbow

Knees

Despite the positive test results, however, I still wasn't sure whether 'True' fibromyalgia was her *real* issue. The main difference between the two can sometimes be the rate and degree to which the body cleans up and improves. While we are getting better at predicting between 'True' and 'Faux' Fibro early in our treatment plans, there are still enough cases that surprise us. I no longer attempt to label one from the other until we are several weeks into the treatment plan.

The misaligned structural pattern Tammy had developed was one of the more common ones found amongst our populace: it's called the *Chronic Sacroiliac Syndrome.*

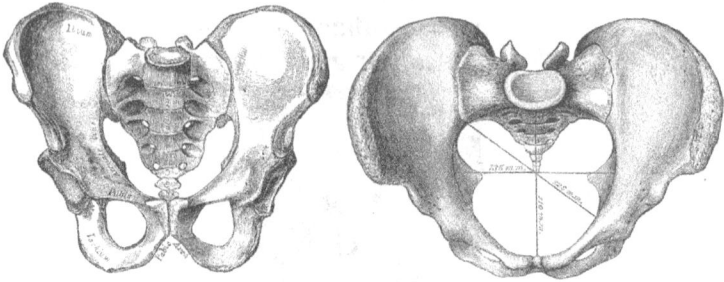

Normal Pelvis

The Chronic Sacroiliac Syndrome

The Chronic Sacroiliac Syndrome (aka 'Faux' or Acquired Fibromyalgia) is an *accumulation* of structural misalignments, creating regional misalignment patterns that accrue from the mishaps and activities of simple, everyday life. While most people understand the need to 'get the front end of their vehicles aligned' now and then, they forget their bodies are subject to the same daily compression forces, yet aren't nearly as durable as the make-up of a car or truck.

What are those forces? Let's start with the everyday, common forces:

The laws of gravity pull earthward constantly on the human body. Over the years, gravity fosters the tendency to pull our bodies downward. In a way, you could say we are compressed from the top downward. That's how grandpa can claim, *"I lost an inch of height as I went through my life."*

Walking on concrete: each heel strike on concrete sends a shock wave traveling up through the body, which then travels back downward, adding – with each step – another nano-meter to the body's compression.

Riding in vehicles as frequently as Americans do adds another dimension to the compression factor. Sustaining miles of the minute vibration while riding in a vehicle quite literally shakes us down like a box of corn flakes. The ongoing compaction accumulates, weakening cartilage fibers and cell walls, leading to the structural equivalent of 'pounding.' Bit-by-bit, minute compression breaks down the vertical tissue of cartilage and advances the dreaded Degenerative Joint Disease (DJD). (And that is before we factor the nutritional dehydration of cartilage.)

Add the effects from any serious structural or traumatic impact as well as the accumulation of the effect of minor daily traumas that happen to each of us every so often: like stubbing a toe or running into a wall or tripping off of a curb or bumping your head on the corner of a cupboard or falling down the stairs or motor vehicle accidents (especially at low speeds). You know, all those crazy things happening now and again in our lives. Those impacts add up, compressing our bodies with every little bump. As a result, Chronic Sacroiliac Syndrome is a compilation of the small physical insults we receive every day, year after year: stooping, bending, stretching, reaching overhead, reaching backward, sitting for hours, settling into one side of our body as we stand or sit, crossing our legs for hours, sitting on a wallet in our back pocket, carrying a purse on the same shoulder every day, leaning on one elbow as we use the opposite arm to write, carrying a child on one hip, cocking our head with a telephone, looking sideways at our computer monitor. Then there are the weekend warrior woes of gardening, cleaning or playing tennis. Those little kinds of <u>every day</u> postural things create, provoke and extend misalignment patterns!

Halves. Halves?

Let's take a short minute for another quick anatomy lesson about the body. Each body has two vertical halves with each side basically mirroring the other. Even your cranium (your skull) has two halves. The two halves of the body are connected. In the back of the body they are connected by your head, spine and sacrum; and in the front of your body by your sternum and pubis.

Your two halves are also connected by five different *crossbars* - or horizontal supports, either muscular or bony.

Goalposts?

Using the analogy of an old-fashioned football goalpost, think of your body for a minute. An ordinary football goalpost has two uprights, correct? Each upright has an inside and an outside.

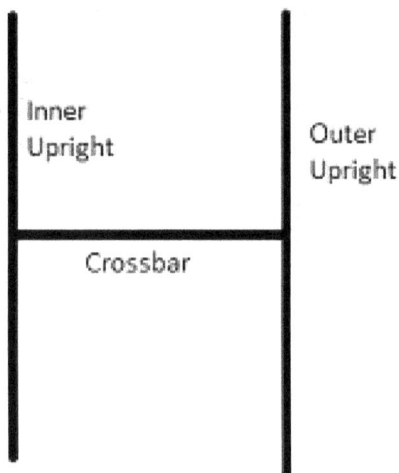

Inner
Upright

Outer
Upright

Crossbar

Your body also has two up-rights: your two legs. Notice the outside border of your body, running up the outside of your leg, over your hip, into your armpit and shoulder?

Notice the inside of your leg as it goes up to where your pelvis begins and then continues upward about an inch lateral to your navel to your sternum, all the way up to your collarbone, there at the start of your neck. Those are your two uprights... the two halves of your body, if you will.

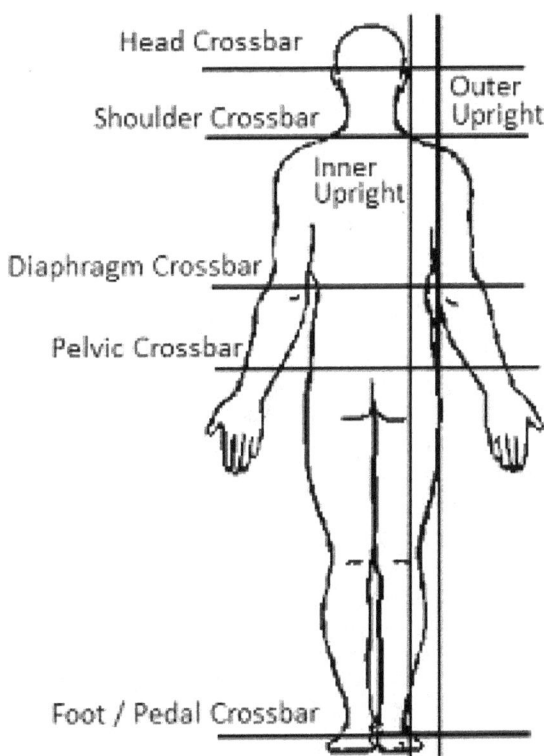

Head Crossbar

Outer Upright

Shoulder Crossbar

Inner Upright

Diaphragm Crossbar

Pelvic Crossbar

Foot / Pedal Crossbar

The Five Crossbars in the body.

Crossbar?

On a football goalpost there is one horizontal crossbar that connects the two uprights.

Your body has **five** crossbars:

1) **At your pelvis,** there is a bony, muscular and soft tissue/ligamentous crossbar. The ligamentous floor of the pelvis is known as your 'perineum' and is attached to the bony pelvic crossbar at the base of the sacrum, all of which is surrounded by muscle.

2) **At your diaphragm,** there is a muscular and ligamentous crossbar (helping to push air in and out of your lungs as you breathe). The diaphragm is the top of the abdominal cavity of your body, housing your major organs, making its positioning critical for the metabolic and digestive workings of your body;

3) **At your shoulders**, there is a bony and ligamentous crossbar.

4) **At your jaws**, there is a bony and ligamentous crossbar. (Yes the area just above the roof of your mouth is actually one of the important weightbearing crossbars for your body.)

5) There is also a divided crossbar **at the *arches* of your feet**. However, the arches are not regarded as a crossbar by all practitioners. It is included here because one of the SOT observations found that when either or both the arches become(s) weakened in any manner, the vertical structural integrity of that side (responsible for the inherent strength of all the crossbars) is compromised.

When any one (or a combination) of the crossbars becomes offset (one from another), the body will begin to develop misalignment patterns. One region will lean one direction with the next region reaching the opposite direction, in an attempt to maintain vertical stability. The offset of those cross bars affects how the body works even in places far distant from the original crimp.

Three of the crossbars are major distribution points for nerve flow in the body. Large, complex and interwoven nerve networks are located behind both of your jaws and just behind your shoulders, on each side of the base of your neck and on both sides of your upper buttocks. The region of the jaw distributes the nerve flow coming from your brain to your lower body; the shoulder areas distribute nerves to your arms and upper chest and the lower plexus further distributes nerve flow to your lower extremities, your genitals and lower abdominal organs.

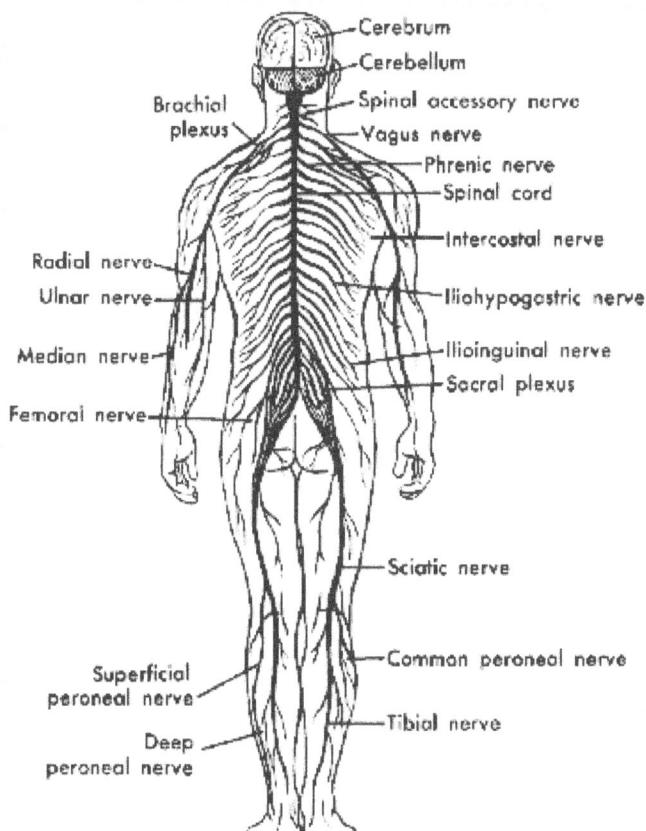

- Cerebrum
- Cerebellum
- Spinal accessory nerve
- Vagus nerve
- Phrenic nerve
- Spinal cord
- Intercostal nerve
- Iliohypogastric nerve
- Ilioinguinal nerve
- Sacral plexus

Brachial plexus

Radial nerve
Ulnar nerve
Median nerve
Femoral nerve

Sciatic nerve
Common peroneal nerve
Superficial peroneal nerve
Tibial nerve
Deep peroneal nerve

Two Halves, huh?

Look at your body in the mirror for a minute: find your sternum (chest bone) and your pelvis.

Do you see the two halves of your body now? The Right and the Left? A bit of variation is normal from side to side. Notice if one shoulder is higher than the other; notice if one knee is higher than the other. Put your hands on your hipbones: is one hip higher than the other? Is one ear higher than the other?

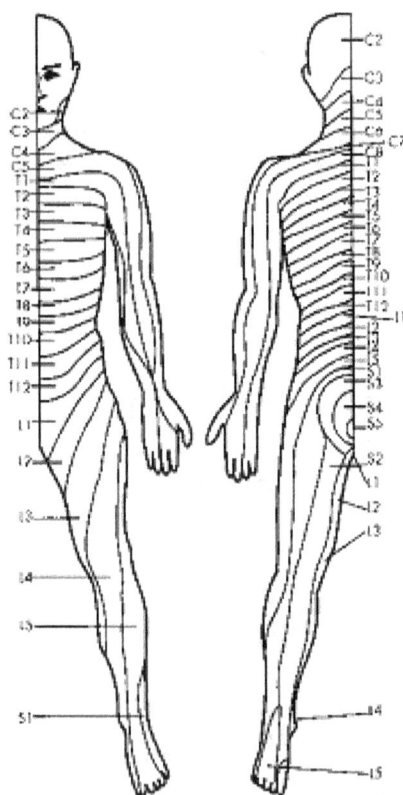

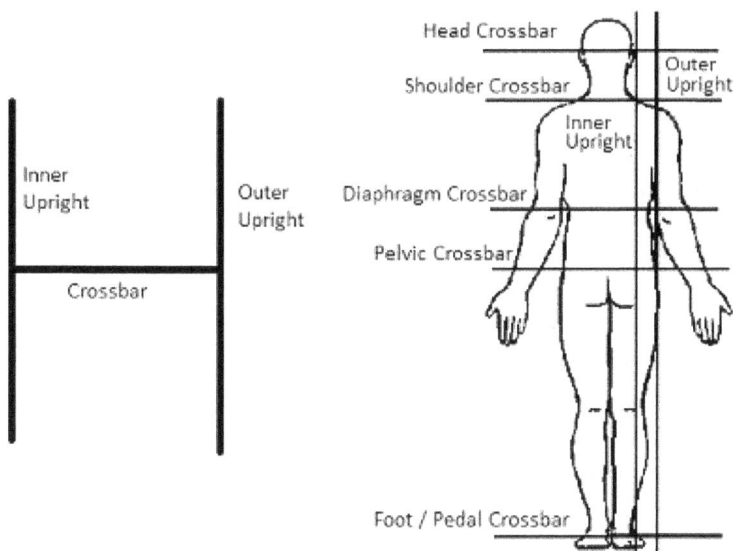

Having the two vertical sides of your body offset, one from another, changes their ability to communicate clearly with each other. That misalignment pattern may be causing you to experience pain between your shoulder blades, stress incontinence, one arm falling asleep sometimes, pain or weakness at your wrist, pain or a sense of weakness or vulnerability at your hips or knees or ankles, headaches or occasional dizziness, or maybe sinus or snoring concerns. All of those are indications of structural dys-integrity and nerve dysfunction. All of those are often components of the Chronic Sacroiliac Syndrome. All of those are often components of fibromyalgia.

With the spine being the common connection between three of the upper four crossbars, one can quickly understand how any spinal and/or pelvic misalignment pattern can torque or offset any one of those crossbars. Couldn't that affect nerve flow in and out and around your abdomen and all of its organs? When several of the crossbars are involved, wouldn't the flattening or stretching or buckling of a nerve due to something such as a lateral curve (scoliosis) or a change due to disease (arthritis) affect or possibly even impede nerve flow both in and out of the spine and brain? Since your power supply determines your energy supply, couldn't the

47

compromised nerve flow of a twisted structure affect the energy output of the body and its parts? How's your energy been lately?

The offset between body halves can change the nerve flow from one half to the other. Our network of nerve systems require all body parts to work together in order for the whole to function as one unit. Can you begin to understand how the power supply to all of your body systems can become compromised when your frame is out of sync?

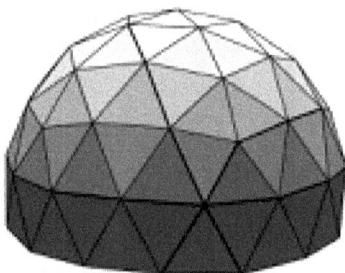

With a decrease in the energy supplied through your spinal nerves, your two vertical sides become compromised in their ability to communicate to one another. This is the first layer of neurological compromise that, over time, provokes a shift of the way the whole body fits together and works together.

Over time, the body ends up with three layers of problem areas:

1) The structural bony parts are misaligning, adding dysfunction and/or pain along the long bony parts with their nerve routes, causing weakness and instability to the compromised neurological function. That can lead to increased pain with further disruptions in digestion and blood circulation.

2) The muscular and soft tissues are starved of their power supply, provoking clumsiness or vulnerability of weakened extremity joints. Added together, you have a body set up for physical trouble, bound for either physical - or metabolic - failure. It is sad to see so many of our elders in this state of compromise and vulnerability.

3) The third may be the most dangerous, and often, the least considered: the cellular changes accompanying chronic com-

pression, distortion or undernourishment of nerve tissue and its surrounding cellular field during the time the body is mis-aligned. Sometimes this down-line destruction (cellulitis, herniated disc, gangrene) can't be regained.

Back To Our Story

For Tammy, the disparity between the two halves of her body was some of the widest I've seen. Her right leg was three quarters of an inch shorter than her left leg. The adaptive, functional, bowing of her spine was almost ten degrees! There was a discrepancy of 1/3" of the two sides of the bone at the back of her head (occiput), an obvious sign of cranial distortion. The chiropractic indicators at her jaw were among the highest I had seen. She carried her left shoulder 3" higher than her right. This degree of disparity can develop mis-alignments at all levels throughout the back and neck, leading to a plethora of muscle aches, pains and tightening trigger points. With this degree of difference, given time, a person is sure to develop down-line structural and organ-related disease problems.

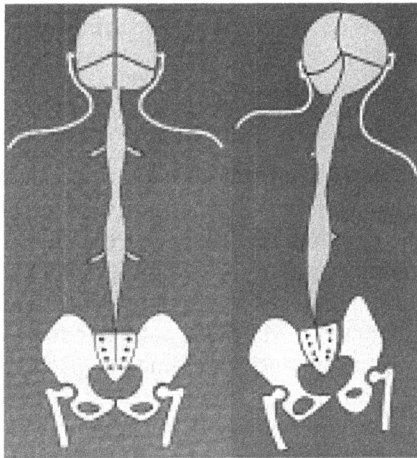

Normal versus Postural Misalignment.

Despite the degree of acquired misalignment, within a day of an initial correction Tammy's headaches were down to 2 on the 10-point pain scale. Within one week she was sleeping, and within

49

three weeks she was waking up feeling rested. Her side-to-side dis-parities were balancing, allowing her pain patterns and trigger points to correct themselves. Within three months, her appoint-ments fell-off because "she was too busy with the kids to come in."

Six months later, during a routine visit, she told me she began to realize she wasn't experiencing sinus problems and she hadn't no-ticed a bruise "in ages." The ability for her to 'pop-out' so completely from such a severe degree of a chronic syndrome – *and in such a short period of time* – tells us she did not have 'True' fibromyalgia. The 18 trigger points that were initially sensitive were due to the degree of her body's inflammation, ignited by the structural torque and tension of muscles and fascia. She was presenting as an expanded case of Chronic Sacroiliac Syndrome. Once all the ten-sion was relieved, once her nutritional base and immune system were strengthened, and once the misalignment patterns were corrected, she no longer had any active trigger points. She had what is known in the community of chiropractic as a Chronic Sacroiliac Syndrome.

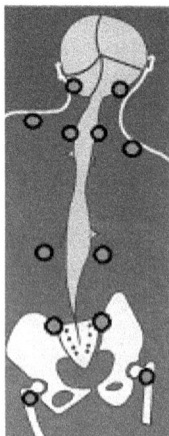

Chronic Sacroiliac Syndrome – What's that Again?

The Chronic Sacroiliac Syndrome is that accumulation of structural misalignments that collectively interfere with normal physiologic functioning of the human body. This syndrome (resulting in pulling, tractioning, spiraling, torquing, or compression of the body fibers) is strong enough to ignite nerve-end-organs called trigger-points. Not all of these misalignments will cause pain, but some can create pain well beyond expectation, and sometimes at parts far distant from the source of the problem.

Calling it a Syndrome tells us there is an *accumulation* of mis-alignments which can include: all or part of the full back (with all of its spinal nerve roots), the pelvis (with its huge dual nerve plex-uses), the knees and feet (with all of their ligament and fascia points), the shoulders and hands (more ligaments and fascia), the neck (ligaments, *nerves* and fascia) and the cranium (where 80% of the human body's neurology exists).

Collectively, the accumulation of misalignments can spiral and tweak the body enough to cause outlying trigger points to tighten and become inflamed, leading to serious pain. Every misalignment needs to be addressed in order for the body to function properly, efficient and calm.

The torque of Chronic Sacroiliac Syndrome tends to start with a pelvic imbalance and end with cranial distortion. Between those two points, the skeleton slowly creeps into a short-arc of spiraled torque. All the while, it promotes a crowding or pulling of soft tissue throughout the entire body. This torquing is distributed throughout the body's fascia, muscles and ligaments, not to mention to nerve-end-organs called trigger points. Many patients tell us they feel as though their shoulders are 'wound up.' They feel wound-up because they are! Trigger points become activated through tension and taut-ness generated by the imbalance of pelvic torque, provoking spiraling of the spine and shoulders. Shoulder and pelvic shift alter the relationship of those two cross bars, changing the way the body parts are able to relate to one another. This shift interferes with the way the pelvic and shoulder crossbars (and everything in between) are able to function together. The longer this structural dys-integrity remains unaddressed, the tighter the spiral becomes and the more degeneration is provoked.

As the spiral twist becomes tighter, the trigger points become more compromised and tender generating a greater amount of neu-ral confusion or neural chaos, not to mention cellular trash, cascading into more inflammation. The greater the amount of nerve chaos, the greater the amount of histaminic cascade as well as pain and tension reflected back into the body.

Unwind the Sacroiliac Syndrome and the trigger points tend to fade.

Ultimately, what those trigger points really define and diagnose is the degree to which the cascade of Chronic Sacroiliac Syndrome has evolved.

Tensegrity

The evolving progression of this structural cascade allows back and spinal weakness to increase. As the body attempts to hold itself up, the misaligned structure cannot carry itself with effectiveness and certainly not with any ease for any length of time.

As the body continues to fatigue in the task of carrying itself around the universe, the trigger points tighten. This balancing concept is not unlike Dr. Buckminster Fuller's concept of Tensegrity, conceptually thought as 'Tensional Integrity' or 'Floating Compression.' As applied to the human body, the theory suggests that the integrity of the skeletal structure requires the maintenance of an appropriate tension and integrity within itself.

In other words, with the vertical structural integrity of the skeletal system slowly shifting off balance, tension within connective (fascial) tissue fibers – starting at points in the spine, on the back of the head, on the back of the pelvic bones and at the middle of both knees and elbows – tighten as a compensation mechanism to aid the body's ability to maintain an upright posture. Known as Trigger Points, these areas are thought to be nerve-end-organs that attach to fibers arising from the spine, pelvis and cranium.

When the skeletal structure *cannot* support itself, the action of tensegrity will cause the tension of the nerve-end-organs and their fibers to tighten, enabling the body enough to at least be able to maintain somewhat of an erect posture and move about the world. Can you begin to appreciate the importance of maintaining the structural integrity of your body? When structural integrity isn't a priority in your health care strategy, daily activities of the world can and will wear down your structure, in spite of good intentions. Your Chiropractic Physician is an important member of your healthcare team.

The Paradigm Shift Component

Medical doctors researching fibromyalgia discover and report inflamed and chaotic nerve actions with congested cardiovascular physiology. They are absolutely right! When trigger points are 'wound up,' nerve and cardiovascular physiology IS mechanically and neurologically congested. As are surrounding tissue and pain receptors.

That physiologic pandemonium provokes the histaminic/prostaglandin and neurotransmitter cascades of the body. This mechanically induced chemical provocation causes nerves to become stimulated and irritated. When nerves get irritated, they DO show bizarre or aberrant behavior – don't you when you get crowded, provoked or compressed? Or chemically irritated?

Take into consideration that when you 'unwind' crowded cellular fields and trigger points the body is able to restore itself to healthy function. By adding chiropractic structural care to remove torques, twists and misalignments, you create mechanical change that softens physiologic congestion. With structural correction added to a treatment program, the neural and histaminic congestion stops cascading, stopping the irritation of pain receptors. Removing mechanical provocation stops the unhealthy chemical reactions. A body begins to relax. The impact of restoring healthy body function by removing misalignments, combined with continually maintaining healthy body function and improving nerve function through chiropractic adjustments is the best-kept secret for living a quality life. Until they experience the miracles structural correction provides, nobody can believe that severe degrees of pain can be tempered so simply.

With the structural-correction approach, the entire chemically abrasive cascade is slowed and can now be neutralized, allowing the nutritional saturation and now-functioning immune system to *really* begin clearing away the residual irritating chemicals. Periodic release of those compressive forces through chiropractic adjusting and manipulation allows continued flow of healing fluids and oils and nutrients into the body's disturbed tissue. Pain goes away and begins to stay away, parts start working, and people start having smiles on their faces. It is heartwarming to watch a person begin to blossom again. It happens in chiropractic offices on a daily basis.

Chronic Sacroiliac Syndrome is not a 'disease.' It IS an accumulation of acquired *structural* misalignment patterns, adding up to full structural stress, sometimes provoking serious pain.

'Faux' Fibromyalgia

At the Fibromyalgia Care Center of Oregon, over 70% of the cases presenting with a pre-existing diagnosis of 'Fibromyalgia" fall into the category of what I'm terming as 'Faux' Fibromyalgia or the Chronic Sacroiliac Syndrome. Each person arrived pre-diagnosed with fibromyalgia, active trigger points and often a history of years' worth of suffering, pain and dysfunction.

Each member of this 70% group walked into our office with severe histories of chronic structural pain and long-active organ dysfunction experienced on numerous levels and spanning varying lengths of time. They were all compromised by classic fibromyalgia symptoms such as low energy, active, real, non-visual pain, multiple trigger points and insomnia, making their daily lives beyond difficult. But instead of suffering from a true disease, they were struggling with symptoms masquerading as disease. Instead of fibromyalgia, we find they are experiencing a severe Chronic Sacroiliac Syndrome consisting of a plethora of structural problems, leading to numerous organic problems.

That says that the problems presented by each person were:

1. Chronic in nature, lasting over 90 days;
2. Structural in nature, involving the sacroiliac and originating with pelvic misalignment that extend through the spine and other crossbars;
3. Multi-faceted syndrome, involving comprise of one or more of the body's systems with multiple symptoms.

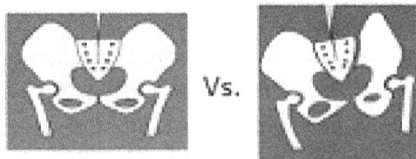

In our experience, bringing a True Fibromyalgia patient to that equitable level of health (or as close to that level as we - and they - can get them) can take upwards of 8 – 15 months.

The economical time of recovery for the faux fibro, chronic sacroiliac syndrome, and/or chronic pain patients speaks strongly to the benefits full-body chiropractic care offers. With this type of chronic pain, a patient would be shortsighted to only participate in the pharmaceutical and medical arenas in an attempt to resolve structural problems.

Until structural problems are corrected, how can you know what is real 'disease' or just a misalignment pattern with nerve chaos? How can you know how well your organs can work until they have the nutritional saturation levels that give them what they *need* to work? Until they work optimally, how do you know what is disease and what is structural chaos?

Another quick anatomy lesson seems appropriate here. Nerves use ligaments and fascia (soft tissue) as roadways to extend into – and quickly communicate with – every cell in the body. Soft tissues wrap around each joint and muscle junction in the body, such as where the neck and shoulders come together or where the spine connects to the pelvis. The joints in the body are filled with abundant nerve organs and networks and other nerve communication. Every joint is a multi-faceted nerve-relay station and fascia is the nerve highway.

Research tells us that ligaments have 10,000 pain receptors per square inch. Ligaments wrap individual muscles and then wrap muscle groups and then wrap bones and muscles together. The interweaving nerves and nerve receptors is a quick and thorough communication network. It works great, until surrounding joints become misaligned.

When imbalances and misalignments distort or pull ligaments, pain receptors are lit-up and cause feelings of pain. By activating pain, the ligament is telling you the joint is struggling, and the misalignment is compromising its nerve power from the joint.

The chronic sacroiliac syndrome encompasses a cascade of misalignments that affect both bony and tissue components throughout the length of the body. By the time enough misalignments have accrued to be able to call this process a syndrome, practically all body regions are involved. It's really a cascading domino effect that accumulates over time with daily life.

Perception Is In The Naming

Not every chiropractor or medical doctor will respond to the term Chronic Sacroiliac Syndrome (CSS). But every chiropractor knows how to correct the numerous components of chronic sacroiliac syndrome; they just may call the components by different names.

Other Names for Chronic Sacroiliac Syndrome		
Pelvic Obliquity	IT Band Tightness	Bell's Palsy
Thoracic Outlet Syndrome	Cervical Brachial Syndrome	Cervical Cranial Syndrome
Carpal Tunnel Syndrome	Trigeminal Neuritis	Piriformis Syndrome
Bicipital Tendonitis	Bursitis	Subluxation
Sprain	Strain	Neuritis

Chronic Sacroiliac Syndrome can also include (although is not limited to):
- bilateral valgus knees (knock-knees)
- stress incontinence
- hip pain
- knee pain
- plantar fasciitis
- flat feet
- mid back pain
- shoulder pain
- AC joint or rotator cuff
- scoliosis
- headache (with or without sinus complications)
- TMJ problems
- snoring problems
- sleep difficulties
- hiatal hernia/acid reflux
- gastrointestinal dysfunctions
- hormonal dysfunctions
- any variety of other organ related syndromes, such as irritable bowel disease or diabetes or gallbladder disease.

What Does The Chronic Sacroiliac Syndrome Look Like?

Let me create a visual for you. During any given school year, as an elementary school teacher writes lessons on the blackboard, she may lean off to one side or to the other, settling her weight onto one leg. Over a semester, as she repeatedly leans during a day, a week or a whole term, she will develop a shift in the balance of her pelvis, that over time will provoke a disparity between the two halves of her body.

The change in leg length is minimal – rarely more than a half-inch, usually only a millimeter or two. One side of her pelvis will become higher than the other. This causes the bone in the middle of the pelvis (the sacrum) to slightly tilt and torque. These changes measure only a nanometer or two in the beginning, however those nanometers can become millimeters and millimeters can make a decided change in how the body is able to perform. Among other things, these measurable disparities traction the surrounding ligaments and other connective tissue, igniting pain receptors and initiating pain patterns throughout the pelvis and its near-by organs. The pain patterns are intermittent at first, but become more and more pronounced as time passes.

Over time, that tilt of the sacrum also causes the teacher's spine to bow and torque as well, affecting her neck. As the spine bows and torques or twists, nerve roots are pulled and tractioned. The cartilage pads between each bone of the spine (called discs) become overstressed and buckled or compressed; they can protrude or even herniate. This combination of actions, creating abnormal wear and tear, sets the stage for degenerative joint disease and arthritis. This is the point when we doctors usually start hearing a patient' first reports of low back pain.

When the spine continues to bow and twist, the shoulder girdle is put off-center, interfering with the teacher's neck positioning. As the neck misalignment pattern becomes involved, doctors begin hearing about problems regarding the arms and hands, carpal tunnel-type syndromes and repetitive-use syndromes. Headaches, hearing problems, snoring and sinus problems often start becoming intermittently active at this level.

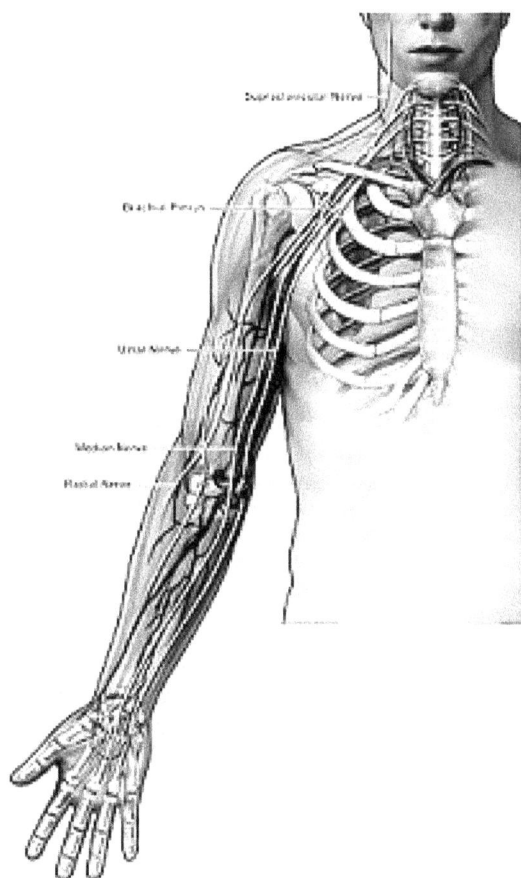

Nerve Map to the Arm (right arm).

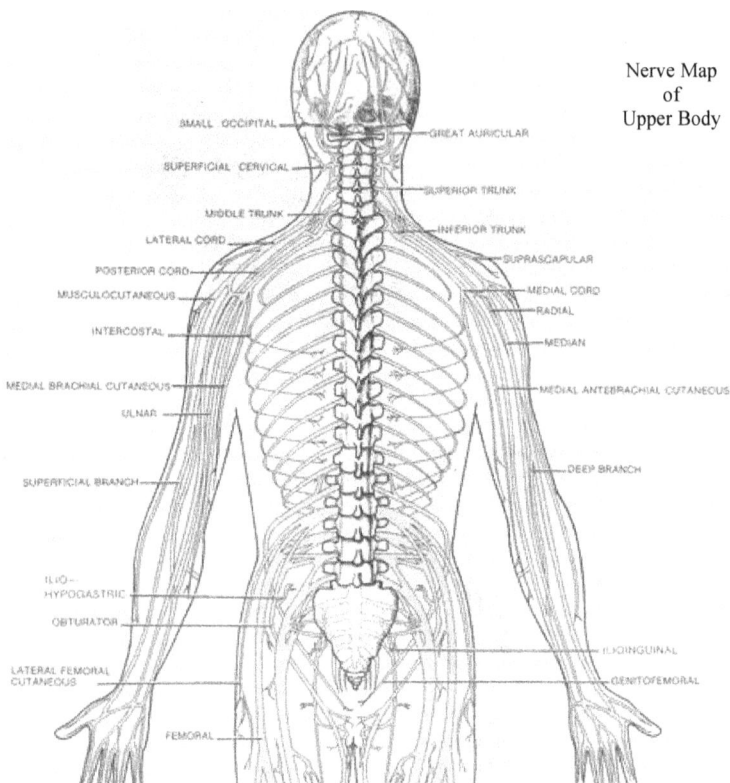

Nerve Map
of
Upper Body

The teacher still has to stoop and bend and reach and write and move about her classroom. Late in the term, as the teacher's structural sacroiliac cascade progresses, her pelvis loses its strength to carry the body. Her head creeps down onto her neck; and her neck sinks into her shoulders. This is called 'turtlizing' and is the start of the Dowager's Hump that women so dread. Turtlizing can be responsible for many types of headaches and neck strain, not to mention spasm, fatigue and weakening of shoulder muscles, and/or increased aching, numbness or tingling in the arms and hands. At this point, intermittent digestive upsets can begin to be part of the picture.

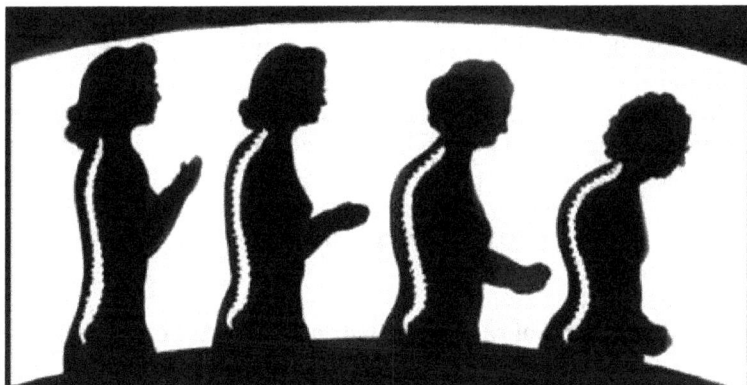

In other words, the neck and shoulders literally join forces to combine nerve and muscular forces to help the *pelvis* carry that person's bodyweight. Talk about increasing shoulder stress! This is when head and neck issues become significantly pronounced. What used to be tight jaws are now *painful* jaws. What used to be occasional headaches become everyday annoyances. Tingling and numbness in the hands become more frequent during this phase of the structural cascade.

All types of headaches, either with or without auras, begin to occur and/or increase at this stage of the sacroiliac cascade. Additionally, sinus problems, snoring problems, sleep problems, balance or vertigo problems all ensue. The understanding I'm hoping to convey here is that these types of conditions are *structural* problems – not 'disease' conditions – and all can often be eliminated and <u>prevented</u> with chiropractic structural corrections.

Tammy

In Tammy's case, each system of her structure was involved with multiple misalignments. Misalignments compromised nerve flow at many junctures. Neural chaos reigned, but her syndrome hadn't progressed far enough for scar tissue to develop. Nor had it begun to involve serious disturbance of the nerve functioning of her organ systems. In her case, avoiding pharmaceutical medications was a very smart choice. That avoidance kept her muscular and connective tissue scarring to a minimum. It also kept any metabolic tendency for toxicity at bay, allowing her inflammation response to be less, thereby decreasing the potential for myofascial scarring. While pharmaceuticals aren't the only thing that can provoke inflammation and pain, the lassitude and immobility pharmaceuticals tend to promote sets up an increase of connective tissue adhesions that physically restrict mobility. The degree of fascial adhesive limitation can be a distinguishing component between 'Faux' Fibromyalgia and 'True' Fibromyalgia.

In other words:
1. Dysfunction of **mechanical** structure affects **neurologic** function.
2. Dysfunction of **neurologic** function affects **metabolic** activity.
3. Dysfunction of the **metabolic** activity affects the **mechanical** structure.
And around the mulberry bush we go!

In this case, appropriate structural and nutritional care chopped the mulberry bush into little pieces. After three months of care Tammy was back in her life. She has periodic difficulties with one particular side of her sacroiliac; but by and large, she is out of our office, moving and grooving through her world!

The Chronic Sacroiliac Syndrome
'Faux' Fibro

The chronic sacroiliac syndrome, (and what I am referring to as 'Faux' Fibro) looks like the following:

It looks like the guy who sits on the wallet in his back pocket.
It looks like the gal who, in order to be comfortable, has to cross her legs at the knees whenever she sits down.
It looks like the person who, unconsciously, leans off on one leg while talking to someone else or while doing some task.
It looks like the person who has that big "beer" belly.
It looks like the person who tends to slump when he or she sits in a chair.
It looks like the person who experiences acid reflux...or indigestion, GERD, esophagitis, Barrett's Esophagus, etc.

It looks like the person who sways from side to side while standing or speaking.

It looks like the person who has diabetes.

It looks like the person who has difficulty sitting in one spot or frequently shifts off to one side or the other, despite being in a comfortable chair.

It looks like the person who experiences bowel or intestinal problems.

It looks like the person with the 'tight IT band.'

It looks like the person who seems to sprain or strain their ankles and/or knees on a semi-frequent basis.

It looks like the person with gallbladder problems.

It looks like the person who tends to avoid exercise.

It looks like the person who has kidney problems.

It looks like the person with sinus problems, especially if it is on a seasonal or chronic basis.

It looks like the person who sits or stands with his or her head frequently cocked to one side or the other.

It looks like the person who has headaches, of any nature.

It looks like the person who has plantar fasciitis or sore feet or heels.

It looks like the person who has lung problems, especially chronic ones.

It looks like the person who has been diagnosed with fibromyalgia.

It looks like the lady who deals with PMS more than once a year.

It looks like a person who has flat feet.

It looks like a person who has carpal tunnel problems.

It looks like the person who had Irritable Bowel Disease.

It looks like the person who has scoliosis.

It looks like a person who deals with pain down the side of their legs or down the back of their legs.

It looks like the person with knee problems.

It looks like the person who had that "gastric heart attack".

It looks like the person with vision problems not related to aging or congenital defects.

It looks like the person with hip problems.

It looks like the person with TMJ problems and/or teeth grinding problems.

It looks like the person who has shoulder problems.

It looks like the person who has experienced a stroke.

It looks like the person who has constipation.

It looks like the person who has osteoarthritis.

It looks like the person who has stress incontinence.

It looks like the person who has a hernia.

It looks like the person who calls himself/herself 'clumsy.'

It looks like the person who has bursitis.

It looks like the person who has a proclivity for biting their cheek when they chew.

It looks like the person who has sleep apnea.

It looks like the person who has ringing in their ears.

It looks like the person who has experienced a heart attack.

It looks like the person with dizziness, even when influenced with pharmaceutical medicines.

It looks like the person who's bothered with bunions.

It looks like the person with a sports injury, especially one that tends to be chronic.

It looks like the person whose knees give way occasionally.

It looks like the person who snores a lot.

It looks like 1,000 variations of these themes.

Does it look like you?

4

The Chronic Sacroiliac Syndrome: Pamela's Version

Pamela Cousens was 46 when she arrived at our office, telling us she'd been diagnosed with fibromyalgia eight years earlier. The pain drawing she gave us would melt the heart of stone gnome.

She had all the classic symptoms: pain everywhere with all the appropriate, tight, inflamed trigger points with all the muscle aches and pains they represent. She was experiencing daily, global headaches with frequent, intermittent dizziness; pain between her shoulder blades she reported as a constant "6 to 7" on the 10-point pain scale; pain at the inside of both her knees increased with every step; her feet were so sore that sometimes she "couldn't walk". She had an ever present sinus infection, rapid heartbeat, anxiety, depression, frequent colds sores, daily indigestion, chronic and frequent bowel up-sets, periodic bouts of bronchitis with other respiratory and immune challenges, sleep disturbances – *all* of which just built more anxiety – not to mention pain, pain, pain, and more pain! She looked older than she was, sitting with the slumped look of having been "beaten down".

Through the previous eight years, she told us she had tried just about every type of therapy available to her: physical therapy, massage therapy, water therapy, meditation, prayer, disassociation, bio-feedback, "multiple, multiple, multiple" varieties and combinations of pharmaceutical medications, often leading to nothing more than "more symptoms". Despite all of these focused attempts of healing, "just about anything" could trigger more pain: lifting as little as a coffee cup, a bad night's sleep, pain shots, overdoing it, not doing it, etc., etc., etc.

"My doctors don't understand that the pain medication doesn't work." The invalidation of being labeled as a "drug seeker" in an effort to "just live her life" had been seriously disturbing to her sense of self-esteem.

With a body weight of over 200 pounds, her diet was somewhat less than stellar. Each day she faithfully drank a half-gallon of water sweetened with NutraSweet at 14 regimented times throughout her day. "I spent years of having my mind so warped I couldn't think." After the gamut of pain medications (including narcotics), one day she made the decision to stop it all. She increased her self-discipline with strict determination to cleanse her system of as much "chemical chaos" as possible.

Choosing to stay as "clean as she could", Pamela was using only *Ibuprofen* or "an occasional *Vistaril*" as her medications. Not yet realizing the need to replace what the chemical chaos has cost her, she was not taking vitamins or minerals or any other type of nutritional supplementation. While it's true that drinking adequate amounts of water can help with daily health and body cleansing, it can be overdone. Without replacing your nutrients, an abundance of water can quite literally dilute your inner environment more and more each day. The dilution can cause your digestive and metabolic systems to struggle, increasing dehydration and undernourishment.

Fatigue Is the First Sign of Dehydration

Pamela's fatigue was palpable.

Reduction of fatigue and production of energy requires *both* water *and* minerals, in order for the body to process the water. Yet her lab studies were, by and large, "within normal range." The lesson here is that your body will do anything and everything it can to "keep the blood stable"... in "homeostasis"... even at the cost of starving your muscle cells. Could that be how muscle spasm is provoked … or disease?

Between her fatigue and the increasing immobility that arises from dehydration (contributing to her increasing stiffness, prompting more pain), she found herself becoming more and more socially isolated every day. The point came when she knew she needed to resolve her condition or it would get the best of her. Every avenue of her life was consumed with pain, dysfunction and inability. Cranky and depressed with pain, she burned through relationships right and left, Increasing her isolation and sense of being lost.

Pain takes a *LOT* of both physical and emotional energy! Chronic pain and fatigue can wear down the best of souls, quickly. Pamela had been dealing with this for eight years now. She was *very* tired!

Testing

A battery of chiropractic, orthopedic and neurologic testing showed Pamela had developed a structural cascade of conditions similar to what we had found with multiple other patients: the accumulation of structural misalignments - at multiple regions throughout the body - collectively known as the Chronic Sacroiliac Syndrome. Indeed, hers was similar to the syndrome described in Chapter 2, but this one was Pamela's version. Every person's version is a bit different. The difference is what determines *that* person's unique set of structural problems, pain patterns and their possible outcomes. The differences result from the way each of us uses our own individual body, the way we refresh and hydrate our bodies (or don't), and the way we treat ourselves or toss our bodies around the universe!

Pamela's version included:
- a short leg with a ½ inch discrepancy,
- a pelvic tilt to the left,
- a tight iliotibial (IT) band on the low side of the pelvis with a mildly stretched, looser one on the high side,
- a lift of her shoulder above the high side of her pelvis, which, over time, gently forced structural changes into her head and neck and knees (areas above and below the pelvic tilt and bowed spine will, over time, reflect the primary region's initial changes):

- a hiatal hernia, with its myriad types of acid reflux and indigestion problems;
- cranial distortion with its myriad sinus, headache, TMJ, and multiple hormonal irregularities;
- daily and weekly bowel disturbances along with various digestion and elimination concerns;
- thyroid, adrenal, and energy concerns underscored by signs and symptoms of multiple mineral deficiencies.
- sleep problems every night. (She wasn't able to metabolize adequate oxygen, as a strong nutritional base is needed in order for the body to process and use adequate oxygen.)
- ligamentous and muscular concerns at each of her problem areas increased the pain with every movement;
- pain, dysfunction and immobility (at one point during her eight years she spent eight months on bed rest!!!
- And pain, pain, pain, each type of pain that goes with each set of problems!

Her state of inflammation was so widespread when she presented to our office - such a pronounced pelvic and spinal torque (twist) - that *all* 18 of her trigger points were lit up! She was *not* a happy camper.

Our Working Diagnosis list included:
- Chronic Sacroiliac Syndrome with full spine, pelvic, cranial, extremity and organ involvement with multi-level spinal segmental dysfunctions (aka multiple regions and levels of misalignments)
- Chronic headache with chronic sinusitis secondary to chronic cranial distortion
- Rule out fibromyalgia of the metabolic type
- Rule out Hiatal Hernia
- Rule out inflammatory bowel disease (secondary to Hiatal Hernia or dairy sensitivity?)

- Rule out dairy sensitivity
- Rule out nutritional deficiencies, especially vitamin D

Pamela presented as a chronic fibromyalgia patient of the metabolic type. She was amongst those few who did not clear up within that 'two-weeks-to-ninety day" period that we were getting so used to and spoiled at experiencing. Ultimately, she did clear up and become pain free but fourteen months past before she was able to claim that state. Her case is shared with you here to illustrate how everyday, ordinary, evolution of misaligned structural problems can ultimately add up to more than just one piece of the puzzle. Fibromyalgia is real. It is not a figment of anybody's imagination. However, we are finding that it may not be a *disease* problem but could actually be a *structural* problem.

When a structural problem is ignored and allowed to progress, and as the stages of pain development and metabolic irregularities progress, it's probable that one (or more) of the abdominal organ(s) will become involved. When you have hormonal problems, you can bet that your head (with its hormonal cross-bar) needs correction! Which organ becomes involved is often determined by the level at which the skeletal spine (and accompanying nerve(s)) is compromised Structural misalignment of an organ prevents it either from 1) functioning well or 2) stimulates the organ to inappropriately perform whatever its task(s) is/are along the path of metabolism. Structural misalignment of an organ prevents it from either 1) functioning well or 2) causes it to inappropriately perform whatever its task is. Structural *correction* of the body *improves* the ability of the organ(s) to work. That's what chiropractic is about: an appropriately functioning structural and metabolic system. This seems to be the piece being ignored when pharmacology alone is used to address a sick-organ concern. Even that pharmacological approach will work better once the structure (and nerve) function is improved!

What is a Sacroiliac Syndrome?

Pamela's list of problems and diagnoses told us they tend to either stem from or include (*and* include?) misalignment-provoked symptoms starting in her pelvis and sacral area, then expanding into her lumbar, thoracic, cervical and cranial areas, while continuing into and throughout her metabolic systems, all of those included with the head, neck, back and organ systems. These misalignment patterns evolve over time as we live through our lives, encountering that occasional rotten food or periodic baseboard or cabinet door corner or fender-bender that tend to unsettle our crossbars. The imbalance of a crossbar has been known to start a cascade of pull and twist or bunching-up throughout our nerve and muscle groups until the dysfunction it provokes can't go any further. At that point, the dysfunction could be labeled as a 'disease' and treated with surgery or some sort of pharmacological input. Those approaches often quiet the concern, but neither addresses the underlying nerve pain and structural dysfunction that a misalignment represents. Allowing it to go unaddressed allows the misalignment to continue to provoke difficulties and pain for the part involved. The misalignment can interfere with the healing from surgical and/or pharmaceutical interventions, sometimes enough to prompt a mis-diagnosis.

Think for a moment how each of us – as we, each day, live our individual lives – is subject to similar forces:

Forces of Life
- Gravity exerts a constant, nanometer-by-nanometer, downward tug on all of our tissues, as we go about and during all of our daily activities. With a million or more variations of 'settlement' occurring with each step and movement, gravity adds to the cellular stress of every day normal movements:
- Walking upright, against gravity, encourages the body, with each step, to settle into itself;

Force
- Wearing heels, wearing no heels: each changes the positioning of your pelvis both within itself and within the skeletal structure, changing the angle of your spine as it rides above your sacrum.
- Walking on concrete: the hardest substance in the world for the human body. *Each* heel strike on concrete creates a

shock wave that compresses the body as it travels upward, and then downward, to minutely compress the spinal structures; this spinal compression can – and does - *accumulate* as we travel through everyday life.

Trauma

- Stepping half-way off a curb
- Having a baby
- Carrying children on our hips twists the pelvis offsides, further torqueing the spine from the bottom up...
- "Carrying the weight of the world on our shoulders"...
- Sleeping in a crimped position
- Being pulled while walking an animal,
- Twisting an ankle, landing on your knee, jamming that hip,
- Stubbing a toe during that late-night trip to the bathroom
- Sitting at your computer for hours
- Bending and twisting in and out of cars
- Driving and/or riding in a car for long periods of time
- Standing up and stooping (repeatedly)
- Loading and unloading of groceries or various other 'loads'
- Leaning over a sink, stove or desk

A list of the forces encountered by each individual human body in any given day can go on and on and on.

That Sacral Shift!

Your sacrum can change your nerve flow, both up and down your spine by the way it fits on your body: The sacrum shifts by the way it fits or rides *with* and *within* your pelvis, both as a component *of* the pelvis and as an individual entity, moving *within* the pelvis by itself. This sacroiliac shift happens in various angles or planes, nanometer by nanometer, building slowly by shifting about in your body in response to the way you move and work your way through your world, advancing your twist or torque, nanometer by nanometer, during any given day.

The slowly advancing compression and/or stretch felt by the nerves and their supporting fibers alter the ability of your proprioceptors, those monitoring nerve-organs, to monitor! A built-up of interference may have already accumulated when you have that next accident or injury, making your recovery more problematic! Consequently, your nerves may not be able to give off – or receive – appropriate nerve signals. Nerve confusion is often interpreted as pain. Do you have nerve confusion?

As the leveling fulcrum of the body, and because the way it directs nerve flow, the sacrum's position *within* your body as an entity of your pelvis – AND its position within your *pelvis* – can often be a determining factor for the strength of your sacroiliac joints which, in turn, can be a predictor for the state of your health and well-being. Since your spine rests on top of your sacrum, positioning of the sacrum will influence the ability of your spine to stand vertically, allowing your nerves to work without intervention. When your sacrum is positioned as it is supposed to be, your spine is better able to appropriately position your spinal nerves, saving them from those crimping or stretching changes that seem to interfere with nerve distribution enough to ignite (more?) pain.

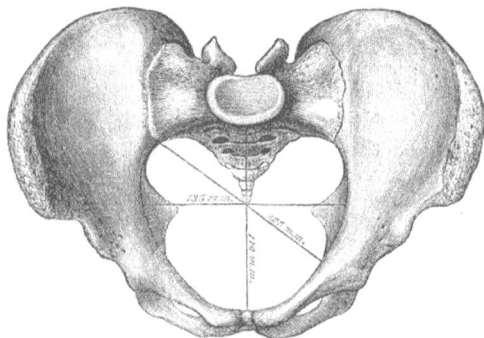

Superior view of the Pelvis

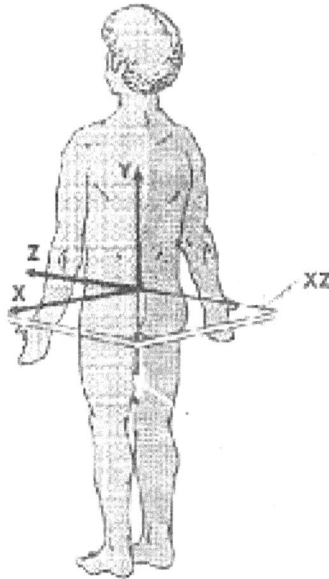

X, Y, Z Axis – Planes of Movement

As well as being the major cross bar of the body, your pelvis and sacrum house the large, two-sided, lower-body nerve centers. Stable positioning of your sacrum allows for stable positioning of your spine and stable positioning of your spine allows for stable nerve supply to all of your body parts! It's beautiful to watch.

You can feel the number of planes of activity your sacrum provides for you: the ability to turn and twist, reach up or down, move left or right, or when executing any combination of those movements. Stabilizing those crossbars both structurally and nutritionally provides both short-term relief and long-term relief throughout your body systems. With the body distorted, movement becomes heavy and awkward, stilted or problematic, not to mention painful and restrictive.

To summarize: Through our daily grind and gravitational existence on planet Earth, our bodies can become misaligned, causing interruption to and chaos within our nervous systems. That disruptive chaos is well known for compounding its way into serious disease! When left untreated, theses misalignment patterns can compromise digestive action enough to create metabolic stress. Correction of your misalignment chaos can change the potential outcome enormously!

Stability.

What a concept!

Could It Really Be That Simple?

You may be VERY surprised. Good health can be as simple as gaining proper healthy alignment while nourishing the body with the vitamins and minerals that are needed to support it.

Since nerves follow all the major bony paths in your body, keeping those crossbars relatively even, one above the other, to the extent possible becomes a smart thing to maintain. Keeping the cross bars as level as is possible within our world of 'walking-on-concrete' and 'riding-in-vehicles' appears to be one of the best things you personally can do to keep nerve flow flowing. Appropriate, body-wide, structural care can align the cross bars, taking the torqued (excitatory) pull off of the trigger points.

Trigger points are activated when crossbars are un-level.

Aquired Fibromyalgia
and
Chronic Sacroialic Sydrome
Trigger/Myofacial Points

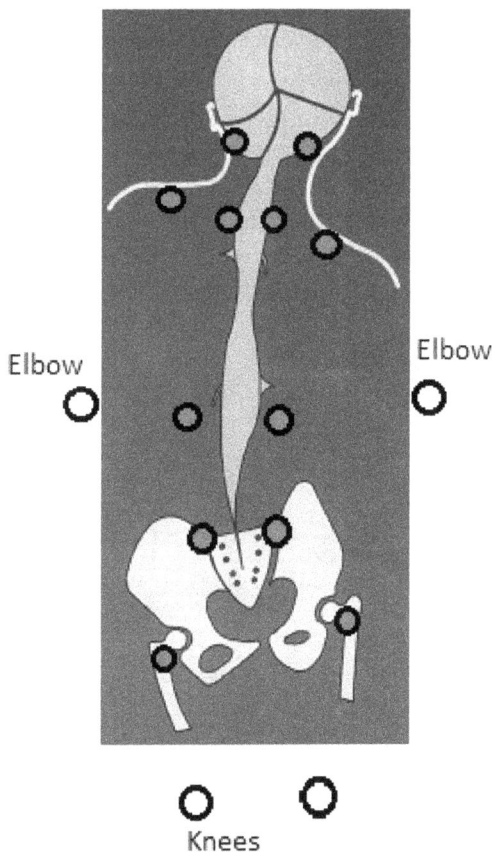

Elbow   Elbow

Knees

Unleveled or tightening trigger points activate nerves and their prostaglandins and neuro-transmitters (nerve juices). Inappropriate or inadequate nutritional levels prevent the neutralization of those juices and their transmitters, releasing their resultant metabolic 'sting'. Some foods accentuate the situation. Pain (with its chemical 'trash') builds and accumulates with your medications unable to fully neutralize or flush the confusion. Can you see how all this can build and add up to *more* pain over time?

This may be clearer with a review of the basic facts about your body:

- Nerves follow all the major bony paths in our bodies... making structural integrity one of our basic needs in order to be able to stand or move in any direction, for any task, including clear thinking!

- The major nerves in our bodies follow all the major bony paths in our bodies...meaning our nerves use our skeleton as a roadway. When skeletal or structural integrity is compromised, nerve flow can't get to *where* it is needed, *when* it is needed!

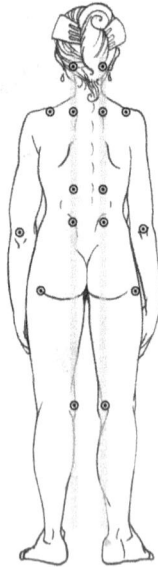

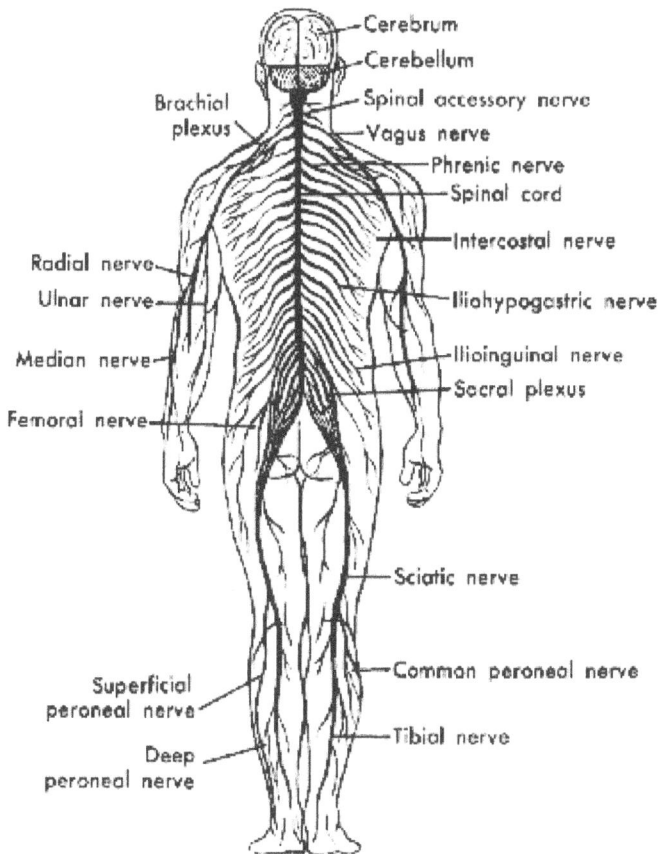

- Each *spinal* nerve serves a 1 – 2 inch-wide area of the body with your powerful nerve impulses traveling the route from the spine to the nerve's end and back. When nerves *don't* work or are infringed upon in some manner, any body part in that one – two inch level can immediately begin to lose power and sputter.

- Each spinal nerve begins by serving a particular section of your torso and or extremities and usually ends by serving one or more abdominal organs.

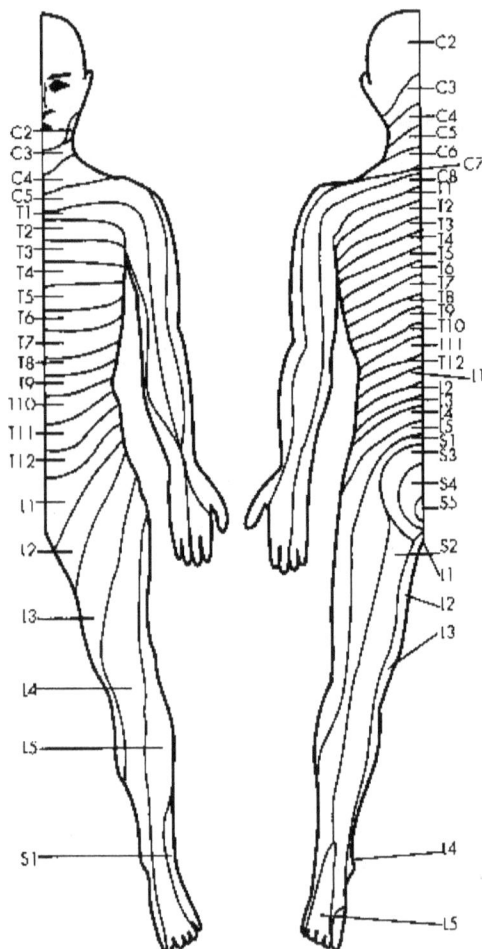

Dermatomes

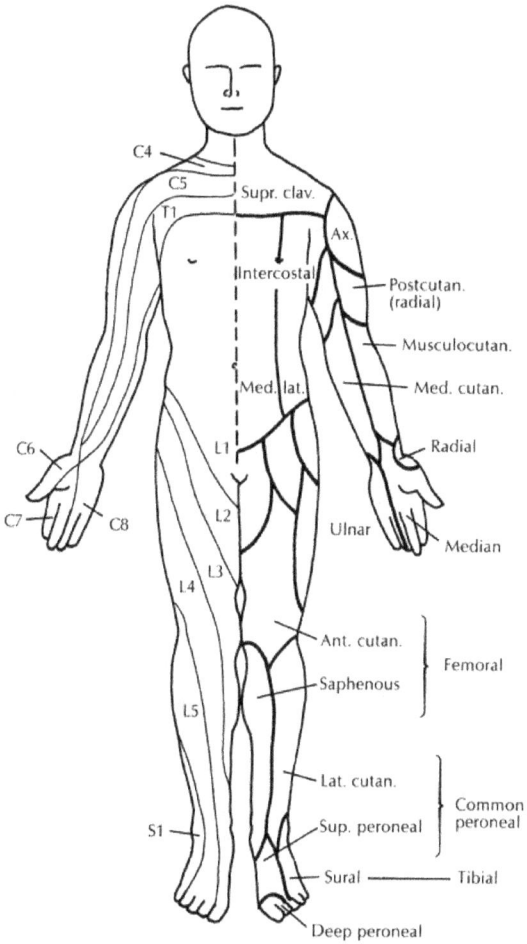

Myotome Map (front view)

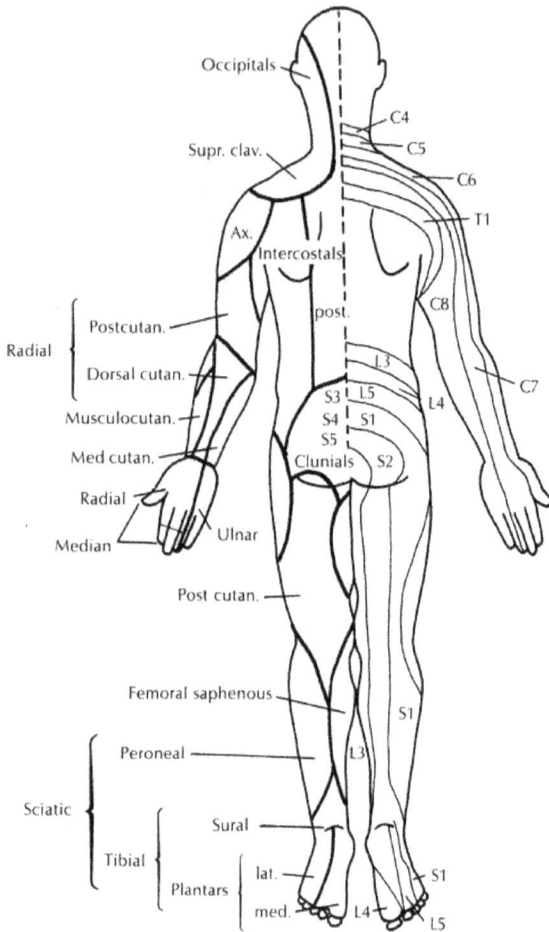

Myotome Map (rear view)

- Nerves serve *every* part and region and organ of our bodies, every minute of every hour of every day. Otherwise, the body (or an area of your body) dies... making full operation of those nerves a minute-by-minute priority in order for your body to function throughout its life. This is why periodic structural correction is such a necessary component in today's health needs. Until you get your body corrected and your nerve flow functioning at its 'make-things-work' level, how do you know what is really compromising your system?

- Each and _every_ joint, throughout the body, serves as a relay station for nerve flow: _each_ joint facilitates the arrival of the nerve impulse to its destination; each joint participates in increasing or decreasing the nerve's power along its path; _each_ joint aids in directing the nerve impulse to the appropriate point or area or destination of need. THIS is the anatomical fact that enables us to understand and appreciate the need for _structural_ correction in disease-resolution and pain- reduction treatment plans.

Nerve Flow Moves The Body!

Consider for a minute how your sacrum acts as the _fulcrum_ of your body, supporting your spine with its rib cage, shoulder girdle and head. Your sacrum has the ability to move both _with_ the pelvis (all three bones moving in tandem) and/or it can move _within_ the pelvis, moving independently between those two side bones. The ability to have both of those areas of motion is what makes the positioning of the sacrum so very important within your structural needs.

This small, triangular bone also aids your body by housing (and protecting) the largest nerve center in your body. Called the Lumbar Plexus, this two-sided nerve distribution center provides nerves for the lower abdomen, pelvis and extremities while also providing nerve-relay-centers and distributing power to our lower abdominal organs, all of our pelvic organs and our lower extremities. All of these vital structures are living and arising in a part of our body that can easily become mechanically disrupted. This mechanical pelvic disruption can affect nerves and nerve flow coming from all points of your structure, creating chaos in your nerve flow, sometimes provoking sudden misdirection of your movements and certainly affecting your hormonal and metabolic activities. Could that be what happens when the cup doesn't quite make the table or a curve ball flies wide of the plate...or you just plain and simply don't have enough energy to get out of bed?

Your sacrum provides the 'stand' for your spine and acts as the distribution center for all of those lower nerves. It is the *base* upon which your spine stands. Ergo, if your pelvis leans off to one side, your spine could be pulled off towards that one side. When the sacrum moves within the pelvis, it can start a twist in the spine that could result in pulling the spine into the curve of a scoliosis... or maybe be the torque that starts or results in the tightening of your trigger points.

Can you see now, how the offside positioning of your sacrum and/or pelvis can lead to mechanical disruption of your nerve (electrical power) supply? Or lead to developing that sudden zinger down the back of your arm to the elbow? Or possibly provoking that sharp pain at your heel when you step down?

Activation of Trigger Points due to Sacral or Pelvic Positioning?

By now, you've realized several new things about your body:

- You've learned about the structural association between your pelvis and your sacrum and you've learned of the relationship between your sacrum and your spine...allowing you to see how the positioning of your sacrum can be affected according to any *pelvic* movement and by any *spinal* movement as well.
- You've learned that the sacrum is the *fulcrum* of your body with your spine being supported by the sacrum.
- You have learned about the five crossbars of the body and the importance of keeping them relatively level though any given day or activity.
- You've learned that nerves use your structure as a road-way and that those nerves 'travel' both ways: to the organ from the spine and from the organ *to* the spine, empowering all the pieces, parts, arteries and veins and organs of your body between here and there and back.

- You've learned about trigger points and how their positioning (and responsiveness) throughout your back, neck, head and upper leg can be affected depending on the positioning of those stabilizing cross-bars.
- You've learned that the five crossbars are assisted to remain parallel according to the positioning of the sacrum, spine and/or pelvis or head.

My Head Is Part Of This Equation

Yes, your *entire* skull with its 23 – 25 bones and 45 – 48 joints and that MAJOR cross-bar can be a significant contributor to your structural stability, your hormonal *availability,* and critical neurotansmitters. You already know your head houses your brain, with all of *its* mighty abilities (and its dozen or so internal brain organs and critical neurotransmitters), along with your twelve cranial nerves (necessary for the functioning of your brain organs)... but did you know that the housing for your thalamus, hypothalamus and pituitary glands (your major hormone-producing organs) are attached to that top-most crossbar in your skull? Doesn't that make its positioning highly influential on your body's ability to produce its necessary hormones and critical neurotransmitters? Does this help you understand how any *structural* disruption of your skull and cranial bowl can be instrumental in influencing production of your hormonal base? A misalignment can hinder those critical organs from feeding your body with the right balance of hormones to keep you feeling good. This is why your chiropractic physician is such an important addition to your health team. There is no pill in the world that can effect that structural change or lift or facilitate the improvement that comes from cranial adjusting.

Your thyroid is located in your mid-neck region, just down-line from your head's nerve supply, *making 4 out of 5 of your major hormone-producing organs dependent on integrity of the nerve flow between your top-most cross-bar and your shoulder cross-bar.* Having all of those critical neurotransmitter-producing glands so influenced by structural positioning may be a new thought to you but does this insight help you understand how the structural integrity of your cranium affects your day-to-day sense of stability *and* wellness? It IS important to correct the structural positioning of your crossbars. The glands don't work well without it!

Structural integrity can and does affect your sleep cycle, your appetite, your weight, your movements, your pain cycles, your bowels and urinating mechanisms, your energy, your mental meanderings, your muscle physiology, your moment-to-moment moods, *all* of your LIFE! Taking all the medicines in the world can't correct structural integrity. This is how structural integrity has such a MAJOR influence on all of those 60+ diseases that so many fibro sufferers seem to experience at one time or another.

Everything Is Affected!

Correcting these cranial structural patterns can make a WORLD of difference to your daily life. Structural and cranial work put a stop to Pamela's headache patterns in the first week she was here. Her sinus problems were gone within 3 weeks and her next spring was a 'joy' of floral fragrances! Temporalmandibular (TMJ) problems are often more correctable (and hold in place) after a lift of that sphenobasilar crossbar. Eating patterns improve with that correction, aiding in many dental, esophagus or stomach concerns. Cranial corrections also make a world of difference to neck vertebra, often slowing and tempering the development of cervical degenerative joint disease.

Putting It All Together - the 3-Dimensional Picture!

Now, begin to layer those three concepts together. You can quickly begin to see how mal-positioning of your body, back, spine and head can lead to the provoked and distorted trigger points, setting off all the havoc they create! Here's where your mind starts to associate the full connection between structural correction and a quiet body. Can it really be true that structural dysfunction and inflammation go hand-in-hand? (Read the next chapter!)

In *this* chapter, you are learning how the *structural* condition promotes the *inflammatory* condition. We rarely find one without the other. If you are reading this book, you are most likely familiar with how quickly the inflammatory state can set off the structural state... now you are learning how the structural state sets off the inflammatory state. Could it be true that correction of the structural state would interrupt the initiation of the inflammatory state?

Over the last several decades, society's mistake with not fostering health appears to have been in believing that a pharmaceutical product can affect a structural problem. The pharmaceutical medicine can certainly *temper* the problem but it will never be able to *correct* it. It may temper the *symptom*, but it will never be able to correct the *structural* component provoking the symptom. Correcting the structural mal-positioning is still the only real, effective, and trustworthy solution for improving the nerve inadequacy. Correcting the structural misalignments to affect the nerve inadequacies has even been known to improve the body's ability to use the *pharmaceutical*!

The trick is to find the chiropractor right for you. (See chapter six for how to go about finding the chiropractor right for you!)

Your Sacro-Iliac Cascade

Changes provoked by the sacro-iliac misalignments can easily extend and magnify your nerve distortion patterns. That torque or twist which misalignment of the sacrum provokes (with its twisting effect on the spine) can, over time, begin to extend the torque or twist up to and even through the shoulder girdle, into your neck, affecting even the shape (and responses) of your skull. Ultimately it can affect your hips, knees and feet! You are not crazy! *All* parts of the body can become involved. It's this 'cascade' quality that allows accumulation of the multiple problems often involved with the fibromyalgia diagnosis. When all systems can or tend to become involved, your basic structure is at the bottom of the problem.

While each of you probably has one region or area causes the most of your symptoms or most easily triggered problems. Like with all repair chores, clean up the basic problem first and the rest of the systems begin to percolate!

Are you beginning to appreciate how the way your *structure* works can determine the way your *metabolism* works? Both your structure and your metabolism are tied together through your nervous system ... and your nervous system is dependent on the integrity of your structure for transportation support... so it can get to where it needs to go when it needs to go there!

Structure Determines Function!

How do you know when your pelvis is misaligned or is your sacrum isn't straight?

Activities or signs that indicate that your pelvis and/or sacrum may be offset:

- o Inability to sit still: moving about in your chair every few minutes, wanting to frequently change positions within a seat, or shifting frequently in your chair, frequently crossing or uncrossing your legs.
- o A need to chew: moving your jaws can loosen the tightness of your head that develops on either side of your jaw. The head plates begin to tighten together in an effort to contribute their ability to assist in carrying the weight of the pelvis. A desire to chew gum can be a sign of this acquired compression.
- o You notice frequent tightness or the start of a headache or pain at the top of your head where your cranial plates come together.
- o Any 'usual' headache pattern begins to nag at you.
- o Increasing or unresolved sinus difficulties of any style.
- o Shifting frequently from one foot to the other: your pelvis tires and each leg or sacral joint tires after a few moments, provoking a need to shift from one leg to the other on a frequent basis.
- o A sense of heaviness at the back of your head or perhaps at your forehead on one side or the other... your head just wants to fall back or to one side on your neck! And it can take less than a breeze sometimes to set off the pain in your head! Your cranial plates may have tightened unevenly, due to the constant nano-pressure from that un-level shoulder cross-bar... or maybe leaning your head into your hands for a bit of time.
- o A sense of heaviness at your low back or especially at your pelvis or sacral area, with or without any extension into your legs or feet.
- o Pain at the largest point of your scoliosis curve is provoked by your pelvic disparity or tilt.

o Any provocation of mid-back pain, especially of a 'panic-attack' nature.

o Provocation of any type of acid-reflux symptoms. Imbalance of the diaphragm crossbar can provoke a hiatal hernia with its multiple varieties of acid-reflux-type symptoms; they have many different names but tend to stem from the same general crossbar imbalance.

o Any cardiac irregularity: imbalance of the diaphragmatic cross-bar can affect the heart or its rhythm. The probability of any fibrillation irregularity involving an imbalance of the crossbars is strong, particularly the diaphragm crossbar. A tilted pelvis can often provoke heart symptoms as it provokes a tilt or imbalance of the diaphragm or shoulder crossbars.

o Any visible 'hump' at the back of your neck. That dowager's hump or buffalo hump is the visible sign that you have been carrying your weight from your shoulders. That compression between your neck spine and your back spine started when your pelvis could no longer carry the weight of your body... the same time your shoulder girdle cross-bar began participating in the carriage of your body through the universe.

o And frequent or unresolved bowel or bladder concerns such as spasticity or pain or irritation or urges.

Creeping Escalation

Over time, multiple, minute derangements of an expanding number of body parts can be seen accumulating. A general pattern of de-rangements can often be seen stemming from an initial pelvic and sacral misalignment. Even without trauma, gradual structural changes can start a pattern of distortion that extends through the spinal column, changing the balance between each individual verte-bra as they march up toward the head. Ultimately, given time or trauma, structural shifts can be found in each region of the body.

With your pelvic cross-bar now off-sides, the shoulder cross-bar will be nudged/forced to lean toward the high side of your pelvis in order for the body to maintain balance.

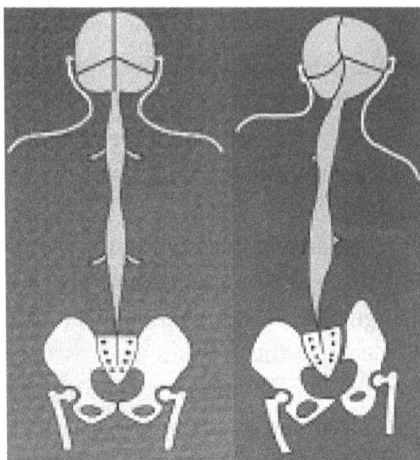

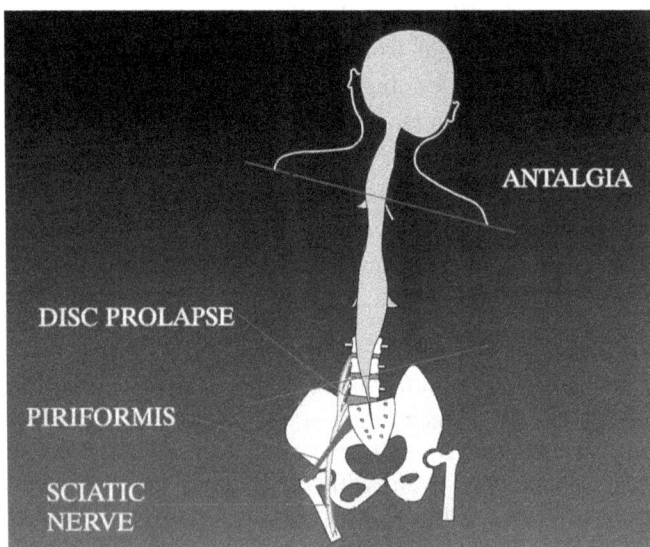

ANTALGIA

DISC PROLAPSE

PIRIFORMIS

SCIATIC
NERVE

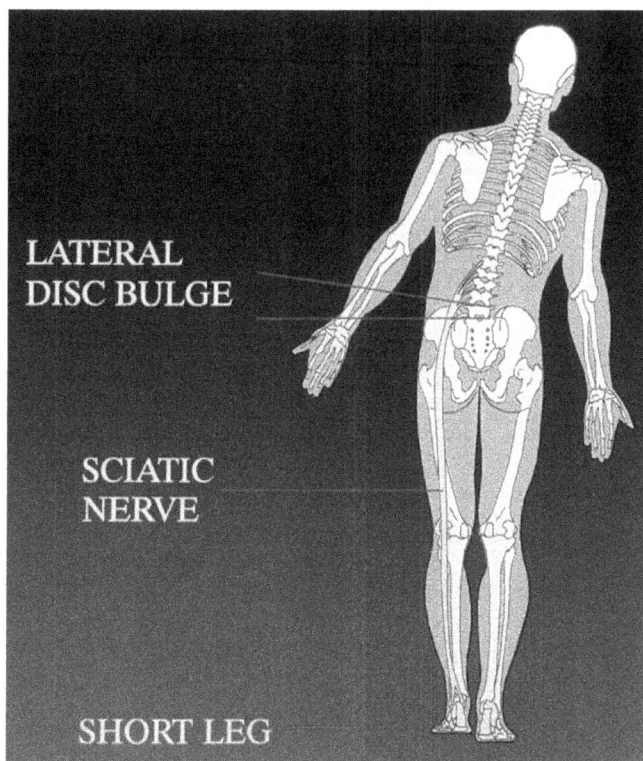

LATERAL
DISC BULGE

SCIATIC
NERVE

SHORT LEG

Exaggerated shoulder carrying the weight: notice the short left leg, the tightening of the sciatic nerve, and the lean to the right.

As the leaning shoulder cross-bar puts tension on the head and neck, pulling their organs into dysfunction, your top-most cross bar – that sphenobasilar bone at your jaws - will add its' ability to carry, tilting your head off in the opposite direction. Visually, this person looks as though they are carrying the weight of the world on their shoulders.

Your Shoulders, Head and Neck
All Start Crowding Together

This gradual, creeping extension of that structural tension throughout your upper body is believed to begin the tightening of your trigger points, expanding their spasms and individual strain throughout their distribution of nerves. Through the musculo-fibrous pull from your spinal bowing, the musculature of your shoulders and neck can begin to tighten and pull together in an effort to assist your body in carrying its own weight. This tightening fosters those trigger-point muscles and connective fibers to cramp, further radiating your pain into your arms, elbows, hands and head.

Your neck can begin to be pulled downward, into your upper body, as it attempts to assist in carrying your body. That crowding together of your spine can ignite pain receptors in your upper neck and across that space between your neck and your head. Due to the increased pull on the nerve networks, your arms, wrists and hands may become more sensitive. A variety of types and styles of head-aches and muscle spasms can begin to develop as your head and neck become involved in your structural changes. You are not crazy. All of those sinus and headache and dizziness issues ARE real. And they are structurally correctable. They arise from structural compression or stretching of your nerves and their supporting ligaments and fibers. That's why the medicines are only partially resolving: the nerves continue to be structurally compressed or stretched. *That* is the part pharmaceuticals are unable to address or correct. Your chiropractor – your *structural* neurologist - could be the most important doctor on your health team!

Got Panic Attacks?

The curvature created by the bowing of your spine puts stress on either side of your distorted spinal curve... as well as all of the nerves, organs, muscle fibers, trigger point fibers and other points in-between. Misalignment patterns slowly expand throughout your structure. Wider and wiser areas and body regions become involved, which is why there is such a varied number of concerns that each fibromyalgia patient may have to conquer. Each offset crossbar opens an avenue for a whole other region of problems to develop.

With that slowly advancing spinal bowing at your mid-back levels, several regions of the neck and back become involved. As the pelvic, diaphragm and shoulder cross-bars begin to curve into or away from one another in order to maintain the upright stability of your body, the power supply for the organs above and below your diaphragm begin to receive intermittent and sputtering nerve flow. That means you experience intermittent and/or broken power supply to those parts. Remember what your car does when the starter sputters? Could that be why (for example) one day you have diarrhea and the next day you can't go?

That intermittent power supply certainly seems to have a lot to do with the development of panic attacks as well.

We watch correction of the thoracic - or mid-back - areas of the spine have a quieting effect on the occurrence and severity of acute panic attacks and chronic patterns of panic attacks. The slight and gradual bowing of your spine changes the stability of your cross bars. This shift in stability can affect the positioning of your back and its nerve supply, which, in some positions, can challenge or provoke the nerve flow of your diaphragm. That sudden spasm causes you to breathe more rapidly, bringing more oxygen into your body, setting off a sense of dizziness, along with that scary numbness and tingling in your hands or fingers.

Those symptoms arise from the rapid intake of oxygen that the spasm of your diaphragm is forcing you to take. It's that rapid intake of oxygen that contributes to making you feel dizzy. A scary panic attack is born... all because of the misalignment patterns of your structure and its spinal nerves immediately above and below your diaphragm. All of which started from the misalignment patterns of your pelvis and your shoulders, gradually coming together to involve your diaphragm and spinal nerves.

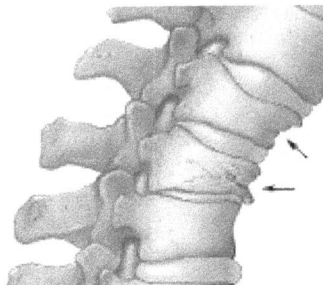

Crowding Towards Collapse and Degeneration

Degenerative Joint Disease (DJD) in the spine.
This image illustrates the end result of thoracic crowding of the vertebrae.

I've taken the time to describe how spinal nerves affect panic at-tacks to give you an example of the extent to which those nerves support and empower your chest and abdominal organs. Nothing in your body happens without your nerve supply... it is the movement (or non-movement) of your body that can determine how much nerve supply you have available.

Once the diaphragm crossbar becomes is un-leveled, all manner of organ dysfunction can and does begin to surface. Inadequate power supplies that the tilted cross-bar represents can provoke multiple types of gastrointestinal symptoms to begin to trouble a person: cramping, pain, inflammation, diarrhea, constipation, block-age, irritability, stasis, spasms, unpredictability...the list of problems can go on through the medical alphabet. Any, and sometimes all, abdominal organs can become involved: liver, gallbladder, stomach, duodenum, colon, appendix, ileocecal valve, any part of your gastro-intestinal tube from your mouth to your anus can become affected when spinal nerves are involved. Which organ become primarily involved often depends on which area of your spine is affected.

Structure determines function.

Too simple a concept, isn't it?

The Average Adjustment

The Average Adjustment for Fibromyalgia Step by Step

At the Fibromyalgia Care Center of Oregon

Many styles of adjusting are available from many practitioners throughout our nation. The following description is what has been found effective for the average cast of fibromyalgia at the Fibromyalgia Care Center of Oregon. Focusing on the general structural pattern as well as including attention to the specific concerns of each person is what has been found to be effective at cleaning the overall patterns most thoroughly, most consistently. What is performed here at the Fibromyalgia Care Center of Oregon is guided by 'indicators' or signs of neurological stress and its effect on cellular tensions.

Patient begins prone:

Step 1: The initial task is to determine the degree of today's structural presentation: is the body pulling on the lumbar spine or is the weight contained to stressing the sacroiliac joints? It is the Temporal Styloid indicator (located on each sides of the head, just inward from the back of your ear lobe) that gives us that information and guides the blocking position. Lumbar problems are blocked face-down and pelvic problems are blocked face-up, each for different lengths of time and with different angulation of the blocks, depending on the patient's specific concern.

Step 2. Three stretches of the lumbar area are completed from the thoracic-lumbar junction to below the sacral base in order to facilitate the stretching, opening and expansion of the fascia and all of its supportive network. The first is directly southward with the second and third being left and south-ward and right and south- ward.

Step 3. Each vertical line of rib heads is adjusted and lifted, from the bottom of the column to the top, addressing each along the way, both right and left.

Step 4. Each vertebra is then individually lifted, starting from L5 and proceeding bottom to top through T1, supporting full expansion of each spinal nerve.

Step 5. A two-sided spinal adjustment stretch is performed at the top of the back where it joins with the neck, giving special attention to that area known as the cervico-thoracic junc-tion – or dowager's hump. It often CAN be eliminated.

Step 6. Wing-bones (scapulas) are adjusted as necessary.

Step 7. Both left and right Calf Sign indicators are checked to de-termine (if any) the degree of the mal-positioning of the sacral base within the pelvis. Resetting the sacral base re-turns the pelvis to acting as a unit rather than three individual structures.

Step 8. The top of both outside strut bones on your lower legs (fibulas) are checked to ensure integrity. Their integrity determines your ability to stand without compromising your knees quite so much. If they are sore, they need to be reset as the lower end of that strut bone impacts on the in-tegrity of your 5th crossbar, the one that is at the feet. Vertical stance on this important strut bone can be critical to the integrity and strength of your lower legs, knees and feet.

Step 9. Both ankles are released and full circular range-of-motion cleared.

Step 10. Each foot bone is checked and adjusted as needed with each toe lengthened and released.

Step 11. When necessary, for decompression of lumbar or facet or spondylolisthesis problems (those of you who have that diagnosis know who you are), Cox Flexion-Distraction is performed at this point, as necessary for the problem be-ing addressed.

Step 12. The bone at the back of the head (the occiput) is check for 'inferiority', meaning: is one side lower than the other? If so, that disparity is corrected. (I've rarely NOT found an inferiority on a person, especially one new to structural care.)

Step 13. This is the point where a person shifts to their back and the pelvic blocking is begun.

Step 14. When the blocking is finished, both knees and hips and pubic disc are adjusted and neurologically strengthened as needed. (Did you know you had a disc as your pubis?!)

Step 15. The Cervical Stair Step and Figure 8 is used to adjust the neck bottom to top and individually as needed.

Step 16. Cervical Spine Lengthening, on the phase of exhalation, when necessary and focusing primarily on fascial planes, opening all those nerve lines.

Step 17. Adjust TMJ bilaterally: this adjustment opening is needed anytime the occiput has been lateralized or drooped off to one side. That sideways pull can pull your bite off, literally, changing the way your teeth fit together. And correcting it can be as easy as getting adjusted!

Step 18. Lift the Sphenobasilar bilaterally. This move is not needed often but I perform it with each new patient and with any complaints of headache, visual or smell or hearing concerns.

Step 19. The cranium is further palpated and adjusted as needed or indicated, checking both parietals, both temporals and the frontal.

Step 20. Both mastoids (the lower outside edges of the bone at the back of your head) are checked for balance. Balancing the mastoids allows the entire cranial bowl to reset, ensuring appropriate range-of-motion of each cranial plate... which encourages synchronization of the sacral-occipital pump.

Step 21. Bilateral shoulders (AC joints) are reset and bicipital tendons released as needed. Each elbow/wrist are scanned for need of adjusting with release performed as necessary.

Step 22. Multiple Organ release as needed and/or indicated with each organ stimulated and/or calmed as required today: Hiatal Hernia, Lungs, Liver, Gallbladder, Pancreas, etc.

This adjustive and corrective 'dance' goes quickly, usually completed within 3 to 8 minutes, depending on how new the case is to us or how inflamed or out-of-whack the person is today. The Cox portions can take the most time. Even then, the adjustment usually goes quickly. It was designed to address concerns of the patient from top to bottom. Through the years we've found, when one piece is ignored or forgotten, it will be the one piece that continues to bark at you till the next adjustment. If (and when) it's all made quiet, you actually can begin to and correct heal. You are no longer guarding against the next attack of pain. This way, you can truly find, get to, your weakest link.

Results of the Average Adjustment

As you can see, by the description of the Average Adjustment, a large amount of nerve function is increased and brightened, starting from the initial adjustment, onward. All three of the two-sided nerve centers are addressed initially, and are checked at each following adjustments. Pain patterns immediately begin to downtrend and continue to diminish! Headache patterns are disipated, sinuses begin to flow and operate, allowing the entire head structure to function synchronously. Balance of the head is restored. The two halves of the brain can fully communicate (what a concept!). And the cranial nerves have full function restored.

5

Acquired Fibromyalgia

"The doctor of the future will give no medicine but interest his patients in the care of the frame and in diet and in the cause and prevention of disease."
~ *Thomas Jefferson*

The immediate change, a decided *downtrend* of pain that structural care achieves, is often a surprise to people. Many people have never experienced pain resolution of that degree without drugs. By correcting the spiral structural pattern and acquired structural defects, cellular stress is removed from the body. The downtrend of nerve stress can often be immediately noticed.

Restoration of nerve function begins with the first adjustment. Sleep begins to improve from the get-go. Balancing the crossbars one with another and correcting nerve action may provide the first instance in several decades for that body to experience full-powered nerve flow. Addressing structural constrictions calm cellular stress on ligaments and organs; the cranial bowl and its multiple nerve messengers are put back into full communication with the brain and the rest of the body; the head is put on straight, balancing the rhythm of the cerebral spinal fluid flow so the nerves and the brain receive the nutrition they need for minute to minute and day to day function. Trigger point pain decreases along with a myriad of other metabolic dysfunctions, improving a little bit more at each subsequent adjustment.

With pain patterns changing and the body starting to function better, the next most immediate and important task is to start feeding it. To *nourish* the body, is to provide adequate *basic nutrients* ensuring that all cellular tissue becomes strong enough for any structural positioning required for *whatever* activity you want to do. Since this nutritional saturation is the slower side of our triangular 3-step approach, it is the next highest priority to be addressed in getting any body back into its life!

Basic cellular nutritional saturation is the next step.

Nutrition? *Yeah, Yeah, Yeah...*

That's the general response most people offer when the word 'nutrition' comes up. Everyone understands the need for it; but not everyone knows just what to do about it or how to go about keeping it simple. Consequently, the tendency to ignore nutritional replacement is strong. It is 'just too much effort.'

Throwing a multi-vitamin at it makes some people think they have 'the problem solved.' We are finding, however, that those tablets don't break down to the degree the advertising may have suggested. Research shows that hard milled tablets provide only approximately 5 to 15% of their content through absorption. They are so tightly packed and bound they are unable to break down, preventing their contents to be available for absorption. We're also finding that the 'plastic,' gelatinous, capsules may not be dissolving to the degree advertised.

It's common to find multivitamin tablets and mineral tablets lying around in the bowel on x-ray films. One study of sewage facilities found that, in a city the size of Tacoma, Washington, residues of as much as 250,000 pounds of undigested vitamin pills were filtered-out of sewage every six weeks. Yes, that number is 'thousands.' Some were so undigested you could read the brand name of the company on the pill.

Despite the 5 to 15% minimal level of absorption, people often tell me how much better they feel when they use their multivitamin.

Can you imagine how much more improved they will feel when they actually obtain 80 to 95% absorption?

What Is Needed?

We review nutritional regimens of new patients prior to starting treatment plans with us. The list and variety of nutritional products they have been using can be extensive. People often tell me they feel overwhelmed, not knowing what to do or how to make choices on this issue. When I first started learning about this side of medicine, I felt the same defeat. However, when you break it down to basics, it is quite doable.

There are **seven basic fundamental nutrients** that the body needs for daily life. While there are hundreds of thousands of other things the body can *use*, these seven are the basic nutrients needed.

The Seven Basic Nutrients
Trace Minerals
Vitamin D
Vitamin C
Vitamin B-Complex
Vitamin A
Vitamin E
Vitamin K

The Magnificent Seven
(With Apologies To The Mirsch Co.)

This group of seven merry marauders contains the antioxidants and electrolytes so often referred to in ads or articles about nutrition. Known as Trace Minerals and Vitamins A, B, C, D, E and K, these basic, fundamental nutrients set-up the actions known as 'metabolism' and 'normal physiology' and 'digestion' throughout your body; allowing 'every day,' automatic, necessary, biochemical functions to occur smoothly, softly, and easily. If your body is dysfunctioning, especially if it's dysfunctioning daily, you could be deficient in several important nutrients.

Look at this list of only some of the every-day interferences that prolonged nutritional deficiencies may cause:

Arthritis * Loss *of Hair* * Leg Weakness * Propensity *for falling* * Fatigue * Toxemia *of Pregnancy* * Sore Tongue * Watery *Eyes* * Anxiety * Arthritis * Macular Degeneration * Blood *Coagulation Dysfunction* * Muscle Pain * Stomach *Burning* * Slow Wound Healing * *Kidney or Gall Bladder Stones* * Slow Metabolism * Constipation * Carpal Tunnel * *Painful Bursae* * Muscle Sensitivity * *Pre- or Peri-menstrual syndrome (PMS)* * Congenital Defects of the heart or brain * *Liver Toxicity* * Low Energy * *Skin itching* * Skin Bumps * *Cataracts* * Inflamed Tongue * *Developmental Delays in Infancy* * Precancerous changes such as Dysplasia * *Petechiae* * Stiffness * *Loss of Hair Color* * Low Blood Sugar * *Gout* * Sores on the lips or tongue * *Poor Ligamentous Integrity* * Anemias * *Eczema* * Infertility * *Osteomalacia* * Autoimmune diseases such as MS, Diabetes, Lupus , etc. * *Atherosclerosis* * Depression * *Waddling Gait* * Osteoporosis * *Seasonal Affective Disorder (SAD)* *

How many of these nutritional deficiencies are you treating with pharmaceutical medications?

Pharmaceuticals Medications

Pharmaceuticals medications need the presence of these seven nutrients in order for your body to be able to even *use* the pharmaceutical medications. People who need pharmaceutical medications – especially if they have needed to use them for a prolonged time – tend to, literally, run out of basic, fundamental nutrients quickly. As you have been learning, a disease process itself can often be the result of decades of structural and nerve stresses, leading to *increased* cellular needs for solid levels of basic, fundamental nutrients. Pharmaceutical medicines, used to treat those disease processes, also need basic nutrients in order to interface or interrelate with the human body. When your body is already so deficient it's in a state of diagnosable disease, the pharmaceuticals will deplete the cellular fields even more, ultimately causing more symptoms, requiring more medication to keep symptoms pacified. A vicious circle! Could that be a reason why there are so many 'adverse effects' or side effects with pharmaceutical interventions?

Therapeutic levels of fundamental nutrition improve healing in a variety of ways. For example, decent levels of vitamin C make a decided difference in the degree and rate of repair of ligaments. Tightening ligamentous patterns is a big step toward stabilizing the chronic sacroiliac syndrome and all of its fall-outs discussed throughout this book.

Through the years, some doctors have told me that tightening ligaments is not possible to do.

"Once the ligament is stretched, it's stretched!" However, with nutritional saturation on a therapeutic level, our patients – or at least the ones who stay compliant with the regime – have found that ligaments *can* and *do* strengthen. That's another reason it becomes so important to develop and maintain a strong *basic* nutritional base along with your adjustment schedule.

Fundamental Nutrition

The term 'fundamental nutrition' implies adequate *cellular* amounts of all of the basic nutrients, including water. All of those trace minerals together with adequate levels of vitamins A, B, C, D, E and K.

Remember the RDA? Recommended Daily Allowance? Scientific research conducted in the first half of the 20th century documented the RDA as the *lowest level* of nutrients needed by the human body on a daily basis. The scientists set out to find what the body basically needed before it falls apart. Meaning, how little can a person take-in every day and not have their teeth falling out? That's a "survivor" allowance of nutrients. It says nothing about what the body needs to be healthy! Wouldn't you rather see your body THRIVE?

When neuromusculoskeletal problems and organ symptoms begin to surface, the body is telling you its nutritional needs are beyond the RDA. The body needs 1) an allowance of nutrients that provides the body the ability to fully function on a *daily* basis; and 2) have enough nutrients left over to allow the body to perform any necessary repair. For a person who's been on the planet for 3 – 6 decades, eating the Standard American Diet, there are usually *thousands* of little repair jobs that haven't been able to be completed due to the low-grade levels of the right nutrients. If the body has already succumbed to disease, initially a greater amount of nutrients is needed.

Don't We Get Everything We Need From Our Foods?

Today's medical marketing of health education is putting out a strong effort to convince Americans they can meet all of their nutrient requirements from the common food supply. It might be possible, IF you run your body according to the RDA levels and have no diagnosable diseases or adverse symptoms. However, given that each mineral doesn't occur naturally in all agricultural regions where food is farmed, the probability of obtaining all your nutrients in even a paleo–type diet is small. Especially if you live in a smoggy or environmentally contaminated area, it is certainly not possible. Add into this equation a body that is already experiencing cellular or organ dysfunction, enough to have a diagnosable disease, and it is not even close to possible to obtain the level of nutrients needed from your food intake alone. You couldn't eat that much food in a whole day!

Even though you can't meet all of your nutrient needs from foods is no reason to ignore the wonderful foods grown in nature. They contain thousands of phytonutrients, some of which have yet to be fully discovered, identified or even named! Fill your body with real foods from our earth, such as plant-based foods, leafy greens, vegetables, and fruits – eat LOTS of plant foods.

Seek It Local

Currently, in our country, there is a push going on to 'eat local' and 'get all your nutrient need from food.' Both goals are excellent. Eating local as much as you can is good for because you are eating fresher foods. It is a good practice for your community, as monies are distributed between you and your neighbors. Less petroleum products are needed for transportation as well.

However, counting on that wonderfully locally grown food to provide all the nutrients your body needs is unrealistic. It probably will provide the RDA of the vitamins and a sprinkling of the minerals. But that is not enough to keep a body healthy. It may keep a body from dying, but not from breaking down due to the continual cellular stress that is often a result of our current chemical and psychological world. The RDA is certainly not enough to support a body in resisting the added stress of neurological compromise from traumatic or acquired structural dysfunctions.

So, in this book, the nutritional amounts we will talk about will be amounts beyond the RDA. Instead, we discuss *thriving* levels of nutrition, not mega-doses, mind you, but *thriving* levels of nutrition.

The Seven Basic Nutrients
Trace Minerals
Vitamin D
Vitamin C
Vitamin B-Complex
Vitamin A
Vitamin E
Vitamin K

Three of the seven basic nutrients are best provided to your body through foods: A, E and K. The others: trace minerals, Vitamin B, Vitamin C and Vitamin D can best be obtained through a combination of food, supplementation and sunshine. While food sources are always a best bet, your body uses so much of these fat and water-soluble nutrients that they are more adequately supplied through supplementation. You just can't eat that much food to keep a solid daily level!

> **Minerals Are The FUNDAMENTAL,**
> ***Fundamental* Component**

What Do Minerals Do For Us?
What Makes Them So Special?

The group of nutrients most *seriously missing* in today's American food supply is the Trace Minerals. Using the word 'trace' to describe these nutrients is somewhat euphemistic, as it makes them sound unnecessary. That couldn't be further from the truth. They are actually *more* essential than vitamins and available only intermittently, throughout the different regions of our Earth's crust. They are not available everywhere on the planet. Which is why it is not fully possible to get everything you need from your foods, especially with an 'eat local' approach.

Trace mineral supplements, as available in the United States, are gathered from ancient <u>plant</u> deposits available in certain areas throughout the United States. They are organic, *plant-derived* minerals. Beware of ocean-sourced products, as the body is often unable to adequately absorb or utilize some of the *in*organic forms of minerals found in that source.

Trace Minerals are the 'electrolytes' and 'antioxidants' so frequently mentioned in advertisements and literature. Five of these organic trace minerals are the electrolytes a medical doctor will focus on any time you need medical intervention or investigation. They include: sodium, potassium, chloride, magnesium and calcium. They are the five with the highest usage in the body, but in order to be fully effective, these five require the support of *all* of the other minerals in the pool of minerals. Many commercial products would have you believing that those five are the only ones you need: avoid being fooled.

<u>All</u> Are Needed For Good Metabolic And Brain Function

An important fact to acknowledge is, whenever you need <u>one</u> nutrient that is part of a group, you need the entire group before you add extra amounts of the specific one. In other words if you're not sleeping well and you need extra calcium, use the whole group of minerals *before* adding calcium. Calcium can't work effectively without the others. And stay with powders or liquids when you purchase mineral products; they absorb more thoroughly and completely.

Minerals work synergistically with themselves, with vitamins, and with numerous other nutrients. In order to do any one biochemical process, it is not unusual to need a half a dozen of various combinations of minerals in order to complete the task. For example, each given step in the Krebs cycle (metabolic process to digest and obtain energy from food) requires 3 to 8 minerals at *twelve* different steps. Of course it's never the same ones in any given step. So, while each mineral is important in its own right, it's the synergism of the whole group together that gives minerals their amazing power and abilities.

Did I Read That Right?
Minerals Are More Important Than Vitamins?

Yes! In other words, **vitamins cannot work without minerals**. Minerals *can* work without vitamins. But **vitamins cannot work without minerals**. Of the two, the **minerals are more important.** There are approximately 60 minerals the human body requires on daily basis.

These are the minerals needed:

Actinium Silver Aluminum, Americium, Argon, Arsenic, Astatine, Gold, Boron, Barium, Beryllium, Bismuth, Bromine, Carbon, Calcium, Cadmium, Cerium, Chlorine, Curium, Cobalt, Chromium, Cesium, Copper, Dysprosium, Erbium, Europium, Fluorine, Iron, Francium, Gallium, Gadolinium, Germanium, Hydrogen, Helium, Hafnium, Mercury, Holmium, Iodine, Indium, Iridium, Potassium, Krypton, Lanthanum, Lithium, Lutetium, Magnesium, Manganese, Molybdenum, Nitrogen, Sodium, Niobium, Neodymium, Neon, Nickel, Neptunium, Oxygen, Osmium, Phosphorus, Protactinium, Lead, Palladium, Promethium, Polonium, Praseodymium, Platinum, Plutonium, Radium, Rubidium, Rhenium, Rhodium, Radon, Ruthenium, Sulfur, Antimony, Scandium, Selenium, Silica, Samarium, Tin, Strontium, Tantalum, Terbium, Technetium, Tellurium, Thorium, Titanium, Thallium, Thulium, Tungsten, Uranium, Vanadium, Xenon, Yttrium, Ytterbium, Zinc, Zirconium.

Incidental Facts and observations about Trace Minerals:

- Look for the label of your trace mineral product to read 'plant sourced' or 'plant derived.' That means it's of a 'plant' or 'organic' nature useful to the human system. Some of these mineral products may come from the ocean, and contain 'inorganic' nutrients that the body either can't take in or shouldn't.

- Through much trial and error, over the years, we have found that *liquid* form is the most *reliably* absorbed form of this supplement. Therefore, it is strongly recommended to use trace minerals in liquid form.

- Whenever you choose a mineral product look for that list of 60 minerals to be printed on the label. Printing that list says the manufacturer is at least *reaching* for the full complement of minerals

- Seek out a mineral product for which the processing company will provide you an assay. An assay is a test where they've taken a bottle from the production line to test it, to confirm that what the manufacturer is claiming is in the bottle, IS in the bottle. Call the company and ask for it. It assures you're getting a reliable product. If a company doesn't have one for you, you may want to buy another brand.

- Dr. Joel Wallach, DVM, ND is the foremost authority about minerals on our planet today. He is to minerals what Linus Pauling, MD is to Vitamin C, even to the point of each having been nominated for a Nobel Prize as a result of the importance of their research discoveries. If you get an opportunity to listen to Dr. Wallach's lecture entitled "Dead Doctors Don't Lie," take the time to listen to it! He's a great speaker and you'll learn so much about what your body's been missing.

- With commercial multivitamins today, even our most sophisticated brands usually have only 9 to 17 of the approximately 60 minerals that the body uses every day. Could this lack of completeness be why we never seem to quite get rid of our underlying disease problems despite a record high rate of supplement intake by our population over the last 20 years?
- What we know about that hard-milled-tablet delivery system – with its poor ability to break down in the body – is that you're probably only getting about 5 to 15% of that already ridiculously low RDA amount! It is rare to see someone using that system walk into my office adequately nourished. Switch to powders and liquid whenever and wherever possible. Your absorption rate increases exponentially!

Don't Get Me Wrong: Vitamins Are Essential

Yes, they ARE essential; but they are unable to work without the presence of trace minerals. Of the two, the minerals are more important. However, your body cannot work without _BOTH_,

What you want to do is just saturate every one of the cellular fields of your body with each and all of the nutrients for about 3 to 18 months. Your body has *thousands* of little tasks that it needs to catch up on, building and repair tasks it hasn't been able to accomplish because it didn't have adequate amounts of basic nutrients to meet the tasks.

Having said that, the average American needs to consume nutrients on a *daily* and *weekly* basis, enough to *saturate* cellular tissue. Certainly anyone who has any diagnosed disease needs to use minerals and vitamins on a daily basis, and to use enough of them to *saturate* cellular tissue.

Remember high school chemistry? "When any one of the ingredients is missing from a chemical process, the chemical process cannot and will not proceed." In the kitchen, if you don't have eggs, you can still make muffins. They'll be heavy but they still edible. In the body, if you don't have a necessary component (such as a needed mineral), the digestive or metabolic process just stops... until the next time that necessary component comes along. When your liver doesn't have any one of the right minerals that it needs, it simply doesn't do that task! Could that be why you feel so toxic? Could that be why you tend to break out in a cold sweat ever so often? Could that be why sometimes it can take several days to recover from the night before, or a day's or *hour's* worth of activity? We've found out it sure seems to have a lot to do with it!

Can you understand now why maintaining consistently strong levels of these nutrients IS in your best interest?

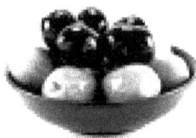

What Do Vitamins Do For Us?

Vitamin C has hundreds of benefits for the human body. Among them is the fact that it provides a very powerful, natural, anti-inflammatory action.

An example of the power of vitamin C involves one of our patients by the name of Doris Brown. This very sweet, older woman had obviously already been crying when she came into our office, bent over with her purse hanging off her elbow. When asked to complete the opening paperwork she broke down in more tears.

"That's why I'm here," she cried, holding her hands out in front of her like claws. "My hands hurt so badly I can't do anything!" She was figuratively on her knees in pain, could not even grip a pen and had no range of motion with her hands at all. The heat emanating from her red-clawed hands could be felt three inches away! She told us she had been like that for two years! Her medical doctors told her they could do anything more to help her. We had to get her inflammation under control.

She began and stayed with the recommended level of liquid nutrition over the next month. Her response to this nutritional approach was amazing! Her body responded to the basic nutrients like a starved child. Removing animal milk products from her food universe had her pain patterns reduced within the week. Her hands and extremity problems stemmed from a close-to classic structural sacroiliac pattern. Adjusting her pelvis, back, neck, arms, wrists and hands helped enormously to restore nerve power to her neck, back and arms.

But, the big turn-around came as she kept the fundamental nutrition into the picture: her sleep improved, her fatigue lightened, and her hands became usable again. The swelling went away, the redness went away, the joint soreness went away, the joint *stiffness* went away; and, with adjusting and nutritional saturation, they stayed away.

Within five months she was back in her life, happy as a clam, and we haven't seen her since. Another example of what can be achieved by correcting the body's structural integrity, giving it what it needs, taking away what causes it to have problems and then getting out of its way and letting it heal itself!

Vitamin C deficiencies cause: Weakness, fatigue, poor appetite, poor/slow growth (height, hair, skin, wound healing, scar breakdown), anemia (unable to absorb iron), swollen, inflamed gums, loosened teeth, retention of fluids, swollen joints, shortness of breath, petechial hemorrhages (pinpoint tiny red spots on the skin), infections easily developed, neurotic disturbances (hypochondrias, depression, hysteria), cataract formation, precancerous tissue changes (cervical dysplasias/ metaplasias), blood vessel plaques (artheriosclerosis), blood cell stickiness/clot formation, sperm agglutination/male infertility.

Vitamin C Actions
- Co-factor necessary for other vitamins' functioning
- Essential for collagen formation and repair of cartilage and discs
- Essential component for red blood cells' production and maturation
- Powerful antioxidant protector
- Aids in fighting off foreign invaders (bacteria, viruses, parasites, yeasts, free radicals)
- Protects against cellular damage (guards against wrinkles)
- Increases oxygen intake, improving the ability for the respiratory system and other cellular fields to function
- Aids in connective tissue formation (healing of fascia)
- Essential in immune system function (protecting against infections)
- Powerful aid to wound healing
- Maintains health bones, teeth and gums (prevents gum disease)
- Forms collagen involved in building/maintaining the health of blood vessels and teeth
- Promotes the development of bones, cartilage (discs), muscle, and blood vessels
- Essential for the absorption of iron and calcium
- Helps to protect fat-soluble vitamins and fatty acids from oxidation
- Neutralizes free radicals and pollutants
- Necessary for production of antibodies to protect against foreign invaders, such as germs
- Powerful, natural antihistamine

Water-Soluble

Vitamin C, like the B vitamins and Trace Minerals, are among the 'water-soluble' nutrients. Meaning: the body doesn't make or store them; they need to be replaced on a *daily* basis. So vitamin C, like B vitamins and Trace Minerals, need to be replaced *every* day. When you drink them, they will be absorbed that day, work in and around your body the next day, and be eliminated within the next day or so, allowing them only about a three-four day life span in your body.

How Much Is Too Much?

Vitamin C will tell you when your body has all it can handle: your body will break down in a short episode of green diarrhea. It's not a bad thing, nor will it be an urgent problem. It's just your body telling you "don't give me anymore today; I can't *process* anymore today!" Being a curious practitioner, as soon as I learned about that reaction, I had to see if I could make it happen, starting the very next day!

Bowel Tolerance

As soon as I awakened the next morning, I started taking 1,000 mg of vitamin C per hour. After five hours, things seem to be accumulating too slowly so I moved it up to 2,000 mg per hour. Using hard-milled tablets, it took 17,000 milligrams in my body to make that green bowel-tolerance action happen!

The *next* day, I went down to 5,000 milligrams per day (which was the amount my studies had taught me was a good solid middle-of-the-road amount for the human body); and I stayed at that level on a daily basis to see how long it would take for my body to saturate and sound off again. Today, with the new vitamin C powders, people often reach cellular saturation within a few weeks, sometimes days.

At 5,000 mg of vitamin C per day - with my minerals - it took <u>14 months</u> (!) for my body to saturate and sound off again! I share that story to provide insight as to how much vitamin C your body actually needs, uses and will handle on a daily basis. (The RDA for vitamin C is 60 mg!)

Down And Dirty Constipation Remedy!

The other side to the action of bowel tolerance is that Vitamin C acts as a super-wonderful remedy for constipation. Bowel-tolerance means when you become constipated, for *whatever* reason, you can load up on vitamin C and poop! We've found it is usually effective within the hour! It is really that easy. No cramping, no urgency… just pooping. But you do need to use powders, not pills or capsules.

The method most effective for relieving constipation is to take **5,000 mg of vitamin C per hour.** Yes, <u>5,000 mg</u> each hour until you poop. It usually takes about 20 – 30 minutes for your body to react. <u>Using powder forms is the *best* way to go</u>. We have found that hard milled tablets take forever to dissolve, and sometimes don't, thereby defeating the purpose.

If you don't poop in the first hour (wait the full hour), take another 5,000 mg. This dose doesn't cause cramping or urgency during your hour's wait; it will simply move your bowels. We've rarely had anyone who needed to go a third hour for a third dosage. But, if you need to, use it a third time.

This is a wonderful, *benign* – meaning no side effects other than pooping – method of solving a potentially serious problem. Using a powder versus the hard milled tablets would make it easier for your body to absorb. You are more likely to have quicker results. This remedy did not work well for people using hard-milled tablets. Instead, stir the powder in juice or water and drink it. If you have tablets, toss them into the blender with a bit of juice. The juice will be tart, just make it a '*so what?*' You need to poop more than worry about juice flavor.

Please, don't allow your body to go more than one day between bowel movements.

By the way, about the color of your urine, the bright neon color everybody believes is about 'too much vitamins.' Bright colored urine is actually the <u>end</u> result of the *usage* of vitamin C and B, rather than excess. It's the <u>end product</u> of the vitamin's usage. Remember, an overage is exhibited by a short episode of green diarrhea. So the color change in urine is the *end result of your body USING the vitamin*, not an overflow of the vitamin.

Change Of Understanding

Using vitamins in dosages beyond the RDA has encountered some occasional resistance, partly due to advertised worries from the AMA about mega doses. Because of its bowel tolerance action, you can see it is literally impossible to become toxic from vitamin C. The latest research reports that people taking vitamin C levels up to the bowel tolerance level and then backing-down by 500 mg, holding that new dosage until the next bowel tolerance sounds off, then backing-down another 500 mg and holding THAT new dosage until the next bowel tolerance event, etc., show improvements in *all areas* of their body systems. Dr. Linus Pauling, the Nobel Prize winner for his research with vitamin C, was using levels at 30,000 – 50,000 mg per day. *That's* what's considered a 'mega-dose.' The 5,000 mg recommended here is far short of that level.

Don't be afraid to work with your body regarding these nutrients. Over a year's time, your body will be much happier with you. You will notice that your body tends to avoid the seasonal difficulties that forever seem to float around. On top of that, your energy will be MUCH improved and your skin will glow.

B Vitamins

B1 (Thiamin), B2 (Riboflavin), B3 (Niacin), B5 (Pantothenic Acid), B6 (Pyroxidine), B9 (Folic Acid) B12 (cyanocobalamin), and B7 (Biotin) are the most commonly known members of the B complex. Folic Acid is also considered a part of the B vitamins and works synergistically with them, meaning it <u>needs</u> <u>their</u> <u>support</u> in order to work with them. And, of course, B vitamins also <u>need</u> the trace minerals in order to be able to fully function.

The RDA dosage for B vitamins is often in micrograms (μg) and/or the level of 1 - 10 milligrams (mg). With neuromuscular skeletal problems (such as the Chronic Sacroiliac Syndrome), a person often needs to go well beyond the RDA. The human body's daily requirements need a level to actually 1) allow the body to operate on a daily basis, and 2) have enough left over to allow the body to perform any necessary repair. Using amounts beyond the RDA level promotes a stronger level of function in the body.

Facts About B Vitamins

- On average, for adults, we find 100 mg a day of B-Complex together with an extra 100 mg of B6 provides a solid base for the daily energy needs and tissue repair. That means each vitamin within the complex is listed at 100 mg (except for Folic Acid: it will most likely be listed at 400 mcg.). The B-Complex includes 100 mg of B6 and you are encouraged to add another 100 mg of B6 as B6 is the vitamin that your body tends to run out of the first. Your nerve and energy power uses B6 with every movement you make, every time you make it. So you want to add just a little bit extra into your formula.

- <u>Menstrual aid</u>: If you are a female still within menstrual years, let me give you this nutritional tip. As soon as you get the inkling that your next period is its the way: add an *additional* tablet of B6 into your morning POWER drink, starting that day and maintain the extra 100 mg dose every day until the period stops. This decreases PMS, possibly eliminating it within one to three cycles! Your body goes under extra stress during that time and just needs a little extra support. Give it to it.

B Vitamins Actions and Deficiencies

B1: Thiamin

- Necessary for nerve action
- Necessary for tissue respiration (the ability of a cell to fundamentally operate)
- Necessary for the metabolism of amino acids and sugars in the brain and fatty tissues
- Necessary for the metabolism of carbohydrates and sugars
- Necessary for the production of energy
- Biological catalyst; co-enzyme; necessary for the functioning of other vitamins

B1 deficiencies cause: nervousness, anxiety, mental confusion, memory loss, muscle weakness, fatigue or paralysis (especially in the extremities), sense of heaviness in the legs, muscle tenderness, emotional instability, depression, loss of appetite, anorexia, loss of interest in daily task, retention of water, and general apathy, cardiac failure, male infertility, beriberi, numbness, loss of appetite, heart failure. A deficiency in all the B vitamins is prominent in any alcoholic situation.

B2: Riboflavin

- Necessary for cellular respiration (the cleaning and oxygenation of individual cells)
- Necessary for production of energy
- Essential for maintaining the mucous membranes throughout the body and skin
- Necessary for the metabolism of carbohydrates, proteins and fats
- Co-Enzyme for other vitamins

B2 deficiencies cause: soreness, cracks or fissures around the lips, the mouth or the tongue, cracked lips, swollen or red/purple tongue, greasy/oily skin, light sensitivity, redness or inflammation of the eyes, swelling of the eyes, corneal ulcerations, anemia, nerve irritability, anxiety, cataract formation.

B3: Niacin
- Necessary for respiratory actions
- Necessary for cellular metabolism of proteins, sugars, and fats
- Essential for maintaining the integrity of nerves throughout the length of the gastrointestinal tract
- Necessary for maintaining the integrity of the nerves to the skin
- Lowers serum cholesterol
- Decreases mental anxiety (calming your brain)
- Decreases mental derangement (helps keep your thoughts straighter)
- Co-enzyme in the metabolism of proteins, carbohydrates and fats

B3 deficiencies cause: muscle weakness, anorexia, indigestion, skin rashes, skin itching, diarrhea, mental derangement, tremors, sore tongue, inflammation of nerves, skin sensitivity, osteoarthritis, pellagra, muscle weakness, loss of appetite, skin ulcers, death.

B5: Pantothenic Acid
- Essential component of vitamin A
- Necessary for the metabolism of proteins, sugars, fats
- Necessary component in the production of cholesterol, hemoglobin, and phospholipids

B5 deficiencies cause: skin itching, skin rash, burning sensations (especially at the feet), pain in the arms and legs, loss of appetite, nausea, indigestion, irritability, sullenness, depression, fainting, tachycardia, increased susceptibility to infections, insomnia, leg cramps.

B6: Pyroxidine

- *Most common vitamin deficiency*
- Co-enzyme for numerous other vitamins and minerals
- Necessary for the metabolism of proteins, sugar, and carbohydrates
- Necessary for the production of energy
- Necessary for the production of neurotransmitters such as epinephrine, norepinephrine, serotonin, histamine
- Essential for liver function
- Essential for nerve conduction (for myelin sheath formation)
- Essential for the maintenance of homeostasis in the brain
- Natural diuretic

B6 deficiencies cause: depression, nausea, vomiting, mouth sores, pain in the wrists and ankles, ataxia, hearing sensitivity, strange head movements, convulsions, increased kidney stone formation, low blood sugar, increased arterial plaqueing, decreased tolerance to MSG, increased susceptibility to infections, PMS, arthritis.

B6 is destroyed with the use of: tuberculosis medicines, birth-control pills, diabetic pharmaceutical medications, alcohol, sterilization of foods such as with milk or milk formulas, antidepressants, hypertension medications.

B9: Folic Acid

- Co-factor for numerous other vitamins and minerals
- Necessary for cellular respiration and metabolism
- Important in the growth of DNA factors
- Essential for cellular division and for transmission of genetic traits
- Necessary for normal growth and development of the human embryo
- Protects against heart disease, Alzheimer's, leukemia and immune system disorders
- Required for the manufacture of enzymes
- Essential for the formation and maturation of red and white blood cells

B9 deficiencies cause: changes in DNA metabolism, changes in cellular formation (especially red and white blood cells, mucous membranes in the gastrointestinal system, reproductive system and nerves), poor growth, anemia, inflamed tongue, gastrointestinal disturbances, irritable bowel disease, spinal cord deformities, heart attack.

B9 requires: B12, intestinal bacteria, minerals.

B12 Cyanocobalamin

- Co-enzyme for numerous digestive and metabolic processes
- Extrinsic factor in the development of digestive enzymes
- Necessary for red blood maturation
- Essential for the normal functioning of all cells

B12 deficiencies cause: pernicious anemia, atherosclerosis, poor structural coordination (can't walk without falling), demyelination of nerves, memory loss, confusion, Alzheimer's dementia, low growth rate, weight loss, wasting, nerve excitability, shortness of breath, dry hair, scaly skin, bleeding gums, sore tongue, loss of appetite, nausea, vomiting, diarrhea, numbness and tingling of the hands and feet, yellowish coloring to skin or eyes

B12 requires: Intrinsic Factor, HCL, calcium and vitamin D for adequate functioning.

Biotin
- o Essential for enzyme activity
- o Co-enzyme for the metabolism of CO_2
- o Co-enzyme for the metabolism of fatty acids
- o Co-enzyme for the metabolism of some amino acids

Biotin deficiencies cause: skin dryness, skin itching, depression, skin sensitivity, tingling in the arms and legs, muscle pain, eye infections, watery eyes, progressive loss of hair and hair color, reddened eyes, "egg-white syndrome".

Biotin requires: good intestinal health.

Fat-Soluble Vitamins

The vitamins the body tends to make and store, include vitamins A, D, E and K. While harder to build up a solid cellular level, they last longer once established.

You will want to add vitamin D to your morning POWER drink *as well as* dedicating time to be IN the sunshine sensibly. Vitamins A, E & K are not intended to be part of your morning POWER drink. Those three are best obtained from your food supply through carrots, green vegetables of any and all kinds, olives and olive oils, nuts, coconut oils and coconut milks. Information about the *fat-soluble* vitamins is added here to complete your understanding of the body's fundamental needs.

Fat Soluble Vitamins Can Not Work without Minerals!

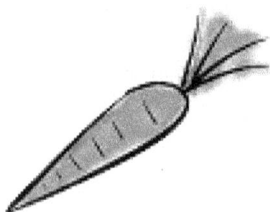

Vitamin A

Whenever possible, it is best for the human body to source fat-soluble nutrients through foods. While not impossible, it is very difficult to become toxic on vitamin A. It's also easier to catch up on vitamin A through foods. Any time you can encourage your body to make its own vitamin, you will get a better, more specific and stronger vitamin for *your* specific body.

A great source of vitamin A is carrot juice: 16-ounces is recommended one to three times per week. It is a wonderful filling food, nicely rich, and wonderfully sweet; it makes a great lunch. If you're a diabetic, use a quarter cup per day and have a 16-ounce glass once per week. You don't want to avoid it – vitamin A deficiency is part of the picture for diabetics. However, you also want to be smart about how your body works. Use the juice wisely. (If you are diabetic, be sure to read the section on coconut water.)

There are some wonderfully sophisticated juicers on the market right now to make your own juice. Or, find the juice companies in your town and use their products. If you have a deli that will make fresh carrot juice for you, have them add a granny smith apple to the carrot juice. It's incredibly delicious.

If you're not into juices, start eating carrots. Assuming you're an average sized adult, one full pound of mini carrots per week would be smart. But you need to eat the *entire pound* yourself, not just 3 or 4 and give the rest to the kids or doggie. Don't slack on yourself with this important nutrient. For humans, red and yellow vegetables and fruits are the best sources of beta-carotene – needed to make vitamin A.

Functions and Uses of Vitamin A
- An essential vitamin, necessary to maintain good health in the human body
- Co-enzyme for other vitamins
- Essential for light reception/vision perception
- Maintains a healthy state within cellular fields
- Necessary for steroid hormone production
- Required for normal reproductive function
- Necessary for normal functioning of the ovaries, testes
- Necessary for the normal production of sperm
- Required for normal development of an embryo and fetus
- Necessary for the growth of healthy bones and teeth
- Prevents night blindness
- Helps eyes adjust from bright to dim light
- Prevents dryness of eyes
- Needed for normal growth
- Necessary for maintenance of healthy skin on all body surfaces, inside and out
- Necessary for integrity of all mucus membranes throughout the body, from the mouth to the anus, including the urinary and reproductive areas, the linings of the respiratory tract and the eyes, nose and throat areas
- Helps the body resist infection
- Necessary for normal immune system function
- Necessary for normal genetic expression
- Necessary for normal overall embryonic development
- Necessary for good brain development in the embryo
- Necessary for human milk production
- Necessary for cellular differentiation
- Necessary for normal, everyday, death, rebirth and maturation of cells
- Healthy cholesterol levels
- Anti-infective against bacteria, viruses, parasites
- Improves skin conditions

- Helps to fade age spots; prevents the formations of lipofuscins or brown spots on skin
- Aids respiratory distress
- Powerful antioxidant
- Prevents damage to DNA

Vitamin A absorption is blocked due to antacids, antibiotics, laxatives, cholesterol-lowering drugs, and fat-free diets.

Vitamin A deficiencies cause: macular degeneration, dry eyes, nausea, irritability, night blindness, blurred vision, eye inflammation, diarrhea, heart disease, coronary artery disease, cancers, poor organ health, such as liver or gallbladder or gastrointestinal problems; crestfallen eyes, low weight babies, damage of the mucous membrane throughout the body (canker sores in your mouth and nose or eyes), tendency toward respiratory or G.I. or urinary tract infections, enhances susceptibility to carcinogens, especially of the skin, lungs, blood or, breast or eye, corneal ulcerations, weight loss, slow wound healing, outer layers of the eyes become dry, thickened and cloudy, causes the skin to become dry and rough (goose flesh), increases the susceptibility to infectious diseases, damages the linings of the gastrointestinal, reproductive and respiratory systems.

Vitamin A requires a healthy gastrointestinal tract environment, adequate body hydration, minerals and other beta-carotenes for full expression.

Vitamin E

Vitamin E is another vitamin that's best to obtain primarily through foods. For good weekly levels, foods can be an abundant and reliable source. Reach for avocados, olives and olive oils, nuts (any kind), coconut oils and coconut milks, and cold-water fishes are all good sources.

Coconut oil and olive oil in your cooking and mixed with your dressings and other foods will increase your E levels. Choose olives and nuts for snacks. Be generous with avocados. They carry wonderful oil for the internal human body and skin. Nut butters are another excellent source for vitamin E. Coldwater fish such as tuna and mackerel and sardines are a good source. Coconut and coconut oil and coconut milks are an excellent source.

Vitamin E Actions
- Enhances the activity of vitamin A
- Protects cellular fields and membranes
- Scavenges free radicals
- Modulates prostaglandin production (protects against pain patterns)
- Inhibits the combining of body substances with oxygen, therefore strong antioxidant

Vitamin E deficiencies cause: *increased sensitivity to pain* (especially in muscles, testes, bursae, and spleen), increased blood coagulation (increasing the potential for heart attack or clotting), fibrocystic breasts, muscular dystrophy, pregnancy toxemia, weakness, difficulty with absorption (celiac disease, cystic fibrosis), leg pain with walking (cramps), miscarriages, anemia, liver dysfunction, PMS, inclination or palsy or any nerve disturbance, suppressed immune system, increased susceptibility to infection, increased tendency to develop brownish pigments on the skin (lipofuscins), hemolytic anemia, especially in newborns.

Vitmin E requires: good liver, good intestinal health.

Vitamin K

This is another vitamin best obtained from your food supply. Dark green vegetables are the best supply of vitamin K. Notice that green vegetables are suggested to be limited for people who use *Coumadin* or other pharmaceutical blood thinning medication because they have such a good supply of vitamin K.

Green leafy vegetables... green leafy vegetables... and more green leafy vegetables will keep you in good supply of this important nutrient. Don't forget your daily dose of minerals so vitamin K can do the job its intended jobs.

Vitamin K Actions

- Cofactor needed for numerous other vitamins and minerals to function
- Essential for blood clotting
- Regulates blood calcium levels

Vitamin K deficiencies cause: poor blood coagulation, cardiac disease, circulatory dysfunction, any disease of the GI tracts that interferes with fat absorption: gallbladder disease, obesity, malabsorption diseases such as celiac disease, diverticulosis, IBS, etc.

Vitamin K requires: a healthy functioning pancreas, liver, gallbladder, and gastro-intestinal health.

Vitamin D

Traditional western medicine is slowly beginning to acknowledge the *vital importance* of vitamin D to the human system. Doctors are finally beginning to understand and appreciate that vitamin D is, quite literally, *essential* for every single process and every single cell in the body. The very best for each body is made at the level of the skin (through exposure to the sun), routed through the kidney, then distributed to every single cell for every process needed to keep body alive and thriving.

Among the *many* healthy bodily processes vitamin D promotes, one of the biggest is enabling the body to absorb calcium. We spend billions of dollars on calcium supplements in an attempt to prevent osteoporosis in our American culture, and then teach our people to stay out of the sun. How much sense does that make? Having been raised 6° north of the equator, on a little island called Pohnpei, in its world of coconut oil and tropical jungles, that '*stay out of the sun*' information from the American Medical Association (AMA) never made sense to me. The sun obviously promotes health. The people I lived with on that island were amongst the strongest, most vital, stalwart people I have encountered, then or since! Sun promotes formation of vitamin D, which promotes absorption of calcium, which promotes organ and bone strength, which promotes sleep, which promotes good spirit, which promotes vital health. At least that's what I watched as a little kid out the South Pacific, and how I remembered the picture, years later, as a chiropractic doctor in the wonderfully green, sun-deprived, state of Oregon.

Vitamin D Deficiency

In Oregon and other northern latitude areas, vitamin D deficiency is common. Yet recent studies reveal that vitamin D deficiencies in Southern California and Florida are almost as common as they are in Oregon. Concerns over melanoma fostered by advertisements from the sunscreen industry have Americans effectively evading any little hint of a sunray on their skin for the last 20+ years! Staying out of the sun, however, is just NOT in our best interest as human beings. Being *smart* about sun exposure IS in our best interest.

Of course, you want to <u>use your common sense about the sun</u>. If you haven't been in the sun for a while, remain in it for only 5 to 15 minutes during the cooler part of the day. Expose your face, arms and chest (30% or more of your body) at least once a day when the sun is out.

When your skin cells are allowed to saturate with the minerals they will have a stronger ability to metabolize the sun's ultraviolet rays. Mineral saturation is absolutely necessary for the skin to be able to transform the UV rays into vitamin D. Without exposure to the sun, the processing of vitamin D becomes distorted and difficult. Have sleep problems? Check your vitamin D levels!

Tanning

Yes, I recommend tanning, both in the sunshine and in tanning beds – though through *natural* sunning whenever possible. Any time you can stimulate your body's production of vitamin D, you obtain a more stable and reliable vitamin for your DNA's specific needs.

If you're in the sun, avoid allowing yourself to burn. When or if your skin starts to become pink, put on a hat or shirt or move, do something to reduce sun exposure! If your skin starts to feel hot, it's time to move or put on a shirt or hat. Be smart. Go get under the trees. Cool off.

- If you like a tanning bed, keep your usage to no more than about 1-3 times a week. Daily usage doesn't give your body time to utilize what it's metabolizing. With fat-soluble vitamins they only need to be stimulated on a several-times-a-week basis, not every day like the water-soluble vitamins.
- Make sure the tanning bulbs are changed in a timely manner. Limit your time accordingly: if the bulbs are new, spend less time than you might if they were aged bulbs. 4 to 20 minutes is often a smart and adequate range. When your skin starts feeling hot, it's time to stop.
- The great benefit with tanning is it simulates absorption of calcium, which is going to make you smarter and wiser and c a l m e r about everything you do for yourself! (Smile!) It will also allow you to sleep SO much better.
- Be smart. Keep your vitamin D levels strong.

Melanoma concerns

For people concerned about melanoma, my recommendations are not an attempt to belittle your worries. There's another part to the melanoma conundrum that isn't often discussed. That's the participation of oils in the dysfunction of skin metabolism that may lead to melanoma. In recent research studies about Vitamin D, it is repeatedly stated that "**a person has a greater risk of melanoma if they stay *out* of the sun than if they have periodic exposure to the sun.**"

In America, Disease Rates Are Sometime Manipulated Through Corporate Mischief

During the 1980s, the American Soybean Association put on a marketing campaign that came out as a national media blitz. Radio and TV ads shouted, "*Don't use coconut oil!*" It was a loud, focused, radio campaign that the American Soybean Association used to garner a greater share of the food oil market. They attributed consumption of the 'saturated fat' of coconut oil to America's heart attacks and strokes and clogged arteries. Coming out of the 70s, Americans learned "saturated fat" in meat were responsible for heart attacks and strokes and clogged arteries, but no one had yet mentioned the saturated fat from *animals* was different than the saturated fat from *plants*. The body becomes diseased from the animal saturated fats, yet *thrives* from saturated fats from plants!

Dr. C. Everett Koop, Surgeon General of the United States, even tried to enter into the discussion. "Your information is incorrect," he told the Soy Bean Association. But their marketing campaign was so loud and so repetitious that his very public comments couldn't be heard amidst their determined message.

Americans bought the concept that coconut and palm oils were harmful to the human system with the result that, almost overnight, they stopped buying product containing those fats. Consequently, almost overnight, the food suppliers and food processors of America stopped using coconut oil. Up to that time, coconut and palm oils had been used in nearly a 50:50 ratio to seed oils (another term for polyunsaturated oils) in our various processed foods. Polyunsaturated oils, such as safflower, sunflower, canola, cottonseed oil, etc., became the only oils used in our food supplies. Over the next 20 years in America, without a balance of the unsaturated oils to the saturated oils, our metabolic systems struggled, resulting in a significant increase in the melanoma and thyroid disease occurrence rates.

Thyroid, Too?

There is an enzyme in the stomach needed to break apart the thyroid molecule in order for it to become activated. Its purpose is to separate T4 from T3 in order to activate T4. An abundance of the polyunsaturated oils prevent that enzyme from existing, so the thyroid hormone has difficulty separating and activating T4. When the ratio of coconut oil to polyunsaturated oil was upset, the body could no longer produce that stomach enzyme and activation of T4 was blocked.

Adding a tablespoon or two of coconut oil a day to your dietary intake restores balanced ratios of saturated to unsaturated oils. The needed stomach enzyme reappears within your metabolism, allowing the thyroid molecule to be activated and, maybe (just maybe, mind you) your personal energy to be restored!

So, you may want to think about looking at the types of oils in your food universe. Adding a tablespoon of saturated coconut oil to your daily food intake, through the use of coconut oils or coconut milks and/or coconut milk products per day, may be a good way to start needed change.

Not The Sun?

The thyroid and melanoma conundrum may not be just a direct sunray problem after all. The vulnerability of the skin starts with a mineral deficiency; over time, and combined with lack of sun exposure, it fosters vitamin D deficiency. Vitamin D deficiency prevents adequate absorption of calcium, perpetuating a whole *cascade* of metabolic disorders like indigestion, sleep problems, depression, decreased immune function and vulnerability to infection. Vitamin D deficiency strongly affects a person's life! Adequate nutrients are vital to life – at least any kind of *quality* of life!

Vitamin D Actions
- Necessary for calcium and phosphorus absorption
- Necessary for calcium/phosphorus/mineral transport around the body
- Essential for normal growth and development of bones, teeth and connective tissues
- Stimulates the metabolic changes in the gastrointestinal system
- Facilitates the body's ability to absorb calcium, phosphorus, and other minerals needed for the growth and development of bones and teeth.
- Protects bone fractures
- Preserves muscle strength
- Promotes brain cell growth, especially for the embryo
- Protects against deadly diseases including Multiple Sclerosis, diabetes and cancer
- Potent force in regulating and promoting cellular growth

Vitamin D Actions (cont.)
- Reduces premenstrual symptoms
- Potent force in strengthening immunity
- Major component of energy metabolism
- Leading player in preventing gum disease and tooth loss
- Signals colon, breast and prostate cells to differentiate into mature forms, to stop growing and eventually succumb to programmed cell death (versus cancer cells that remain immature, and rapidly divide)
- Can reduce the PSA marker for prostate cancer

Vitamin D deficiencies cause: seasonal affective disorder; poor structural growth; dental cavities; poor bone strength; poor ligamentous integrity; slow metabolism (obesity, constipation); restlessness; profuse sweating; delayed tooth development; Pidgeon crest at the chest; waddling gait; sweating; muscle cramps; atherosclerosis; accelerated bone loss; muscle weakness; an increased risk of falls among the elderly; decreased resistance against influenza and other types of infection; increased risk of developing cancer and certain autoimmune diseases; leg weakness (possible resulting in falls); late teething; osteomalacia (softening of bone due to decrease of calcium, phosphorus content, Increased parathyroid hormone; autoimmune diseases; the hormone/vitamin inactivates killer-T-lymphocytes that drive autoimmune diseases such a MS, lupus, diabetes, organ rejection; cellular immaturity and dysfunctioning; Growth retardation; skeletal deformities and anomalies; development of hypertension, diabetes and metabolic syndromes and obesity; cholesterol problems (cholesterol is needed to synthesize vitamin D).

Vitmain D sources: sun, ultraviolet absorption, nutrients that protect and support the skin, liquid minerals, coconut oil, some cold water fish. Exposure to the UV light from the sun is the best option for vitamin D production.

Vitamin D Toxicity And Dosage

As with vitamin A, it's almost impossible for the adult human being to become toxic due to too much vitamin D. Only one person we know actually did and he was Mr. Gary Null, author of *Death by Medicine*, the highly referenced exposé of the number of adverse events occurring due to pharmaceutical medicine in our country. He set out consciously to challenge our knowledge about the possibility of vitamin D toxicity by taking increasing amounts every day. It took him over *1 million international units (IU's) per day* to become sick. *THAT* is an extreme case!

All Seven Groups Are Needed

Having just read about the incredible support these seven nutrients provide for you and learned how nasty things can become in your body when they are deficient, you can understand how nutritional doctors say you cannot do without *any one* of those nutrients. Each and every mineral and vitamin is needed in each of our bodies every minute of every day. It is not a surprise to me that our skin gets thin, or our discs lose their height, dry and crack. Through the years, we become so nutritionally deficient we wither away! How many pharmaceutical medicines are you taking for conditions that could actually be mineral or vitamin deficiencies?

NOTE: as you begin this type of nutritional replacement program, do not discontinue your pharmaceutical medicine regimen. Once your body has had time to saturate and improve its performance, talk with your medical doctor about reassessing your needs. Be sure to work with your doctor for any needed change of your medications.

We all get a new body every seven years. But if we keep doing the same old things, we'll grow the same old body. Nutrients strengthen and improve body tissue throughout all of its systems! Learn to use your nutrients at a therapeutic level if you truly want your body to thrive, change and behave. Get a NEW body!

So How Do I Put All Of This Together?
And Is *'Keeping It Simple'* Too Much To Ask?

Yes! There is a way to put it all together AND keep it simple! The solution? Five little bottles of nutrients, a blender, a stack of paper cups, and 60 seconds a day!

We call it our morning POWER drink! It has made tremendous differences in the lives of many of our patients and their families.

Aren't We Supposed To Space-out
Our Nutrients Throughout A Day?

There have been many patients who feel that way. They felt they needed to strive for that steady, homeostatic, blood flow. What they found is the *cellular* levels need to be kept saturated.

Over the years and with hundreds of patients, it has been found that having a full blast of nutrients in the morning gets the body's juices going and glowing. Then, a drink of refreshing water periodically throughout the day can KEEP them flowing. **It appears to be more beneficial to get all of your day's needs at once rather than to miss half of each day's needs by forgetting a second or third or fourth dosage because life gets too busy.**

Five Bottles?

To get all those wonderful nutrients, **it only takes five bottles:**

 * A bottle of your liquid Trace Minerals
  * A jar of powdered vitamin C
   * A bottle of B complex (soft tablets)
    *A bottle of B6 (soft tablets)
     *And a bottle of liquid vitamin D3

Put them right next to your blender. Add a stack of paper cups. That way, as you head out the door on your way to work with your POWER drink, you don't even have to bring home the cup!

Those five bottles will provide ALL of your trace minerals, vitamin C, the crucial B vitamins and the essential vitamin D needed to get your body revving. For vitamin A, E and K, add carrots (one pound of mini carrots per week), olives and/or olive oil or avocados, coconut oil, nuts and lots of green veggies to your daily and weekly food and snack menu.

This quick little habit can provide one of the best pieces of health insurance coverage around, not to mention cheapest!

Tablets & Capsules Or Powders & Liquids?

Looking into the sewage waste may not be the first research tool the average person would consider, but a recent analysis of sewage residue is enlightening. Testing at state sewage plants has shown an increasing amount of multi-vitamin pill residue in community wastewaters. Turns out, those minerals and vitamin pills we've been ingesting appear not to be breaking down. They are also being observed – before elimination and still solid – on x-ray films, as they s l o w l y pass through the intestines, at best, contributing merely 5 – 15% of what you'd expect to receive.

The lesson here is to eliminate as many barriers between you and the nutrient compound as is possible. This one little change will **increase your absorption** of those nutrients **up to 80 – 95%!** Break up hard-milled tablets; pull apart capsules; pierce liquid-filled capsules and drain into your blender (and don't buy them again). You will actually get more of a bang for your buck with liquids and powders.

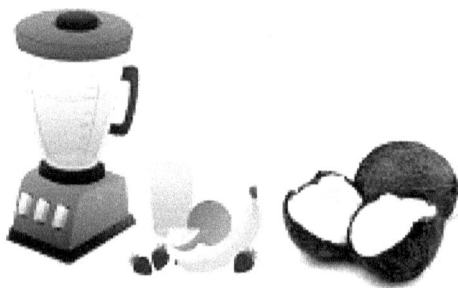

To Create Your Morning POWER Drink, Follow This Very Simple Five-Step Process

STEP 1:	Put your favorite juice, water or coconut water into the blender.
STEP 2:	Add your dose from each of the five bottles of vitamins and minerals.
STEP 3:	Add anything else you want to have for your daily-preferred nutrient or pharmaceutical intake, *except* your fiber. Avoid adding fruits and vegetables, at least initially, as they can bind the nutrients, robbing you of their value.
STEP 4:	Put the lid on the blender and blend for 10-15 seconds.
STEP 5:	Pour into a paper cup. Drink it now or take it with you. You don't even have to bring the cup home!

You are out the door within 60 – 90 seconds with a tasty drink containing everything your body needs to keep you running smoothly through that day with your energy feeling strong and solid. Using this at the top half of the day seems best as when I have used it later in the day, it interfered with my sleep.

Why Is Coconut Water So Strongly Suggested For The Morning POWER Drink?

What makes coconut water so beneficial?
- It has less calories and carbohydrates than juice.
- The saturated fats in it have 1/3 less calories (6-7 per gram) than the poly-unsaturated fats (9 per gram).
- The Medium Chain Fatty Acids (MCFA's) in the oil of coconut products aids in neutralizing polyunsaturated fatty acids, regulating and *normalizing cholesterol naturally*, putting coconut products high on the list of beneficial antioxidants.

- The calorie difference allows frequent consumption to facilitate low-grade monthly weight loss. The 'higher octane' of coconut oils contained in coconut water improves metabolism; 1 – 3 pounds of weight loss per month has been demonstrated.
- The cellular cleansing it provides can ultimately improve insulin resistance, balancing blood sugar.
- Aids oxygenation of the cells, allowing for an ease of breathing, increasing the body's ability to utilize oxygen.
- Coconut water improves the lungs ability to utilize and metabolize oxygen, improving any type of lung congestion. It's a good source of vitamin E.
- Improving the ability of the body to utilize oxygen lowers stress on all body systems, eases anxiety, cardiovascular and adrenal stress.
- It increases the number and activity of mitochondria (your energy producing organs) in muscles, increasing the body's ability to manufacture and distribute the energy molecules of ATP.
- Its antioxidant ability lightens age spots by improving the outer layers of your skin and hair, bringing you closer to your 'youthful glow.'
- Antioxidant abilities protect against aging of the brain, as coconut products are known to temper nerve cell degeneration in the brain, possibly slowing or deterring Alzheimer's and Parkinson's type conditions. Tempering nerve cell degeneration is also noted in the extremities for conditions such as Multiple Sclerosis and Muscular Dystrophy.
- Contains a *powerful* natural antibiotic, effective against viruses and bacteria and yeasts, making it an important medicinal food for Hepatitis, HIV, Herpes, Candida and many types of infections. Current commercial products of this incredible antibiotic property include Monolaurin and Lauricidin.

Important note for tummy upset: If you ever get a little bit of tummy upset with the morning POWER drink, it's most likely going to be the B complex vitamins giving you the problem. It could be the bottle is out of date or you have a brand that may not have undergone good quality control during its production. If adding a bit of food to the picture doesn't resolve the problem, buy another brand at your next bottle. To solve the problem at this point, use a juice that has a bit of pulp to it, perhaps, like a pineapple or apricot juice, to prevent the sense of stomach churn. Or use the coconut water. Give the drink an extra few seconds of 'blend' to make sure it is all broken up.

Promoting the Body's Usage Of
All Those Great Nutrients: Distribution

Throughout the rest of your day, your body's task is <u>distribute</u> all of the great nutrients throughout the cellular field... into your organs, extremities, brain and the cells of blood vessels and glands and parts that need them for daily functioning. The best 'medium' or liquid for that is water. Sipping at water throughout a day is more hydrating than you may think.

Why Water?

The breakdown most Americans equate with the term "arthritis" seems to stem largely from accumulated affects of poor hydration - or poor water saturation - throughout life. Just as oil in a car engine becomes sludge when it goes without being changed for long periods of time, so do the fluids of the body become sludge when they are not frequently changed. As fluids of the body become dense and thick - as happens from eating and drinking the standard American diet - our cartilage cells stagnate and scar, becoming unable to hold the disc or cartilage pad fully upright. Fibrous tissue become thickened and aren't able to hold as much weight or respond to movement as quickly and thoroughly. The discs begin to bend, break down, split, separate and protrude around their edges. Strength of cartilage is dependent upon its ability to maintain its upright cellular integrity, which is dependent on the water levels stored within cells. When cells lose their hydration, breakdowns cause a bulge of the cartilage disc. They take on the characteristics of a dried-up riverbed where a crack or fissure may allow the center core to ooze out, signifying full herniation. The side of the herniation is determined by the direction – and degree – of the spiral of

Chronic Sacroiliac Syndrome. *That's* why water is so important in the picture of structural integrity.

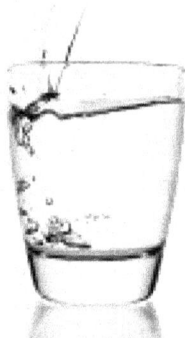

Water saturation of cartilage takes three things: water, minerals and exercise. As cellular storage of water ebbs in the cartilage, those pads and joint surfaces thin, becoming scratchy and ratchety. They have difficulty moving and start to become irritated and inflamed. Pain increases. Pain stops coming and going – it starts coming and *staying*!

The standard American diet with inadequate nutrition and hydration contributes to the development of Chronic Sacroiliac Syndrome.

Artificial teas, sodas and other drink products on the market contain many dissolved food particles. Nearly all of the water contained in artificial drink products is used to process its food particles out of your body. This leaves minimal amounts of water for you or your cells to use. Your cells are left swimming around in *sludgy* potty water! That state is not going to generate a lot of energy! **The first sign of dehydration is fatigue!** Best bet: drink plenty of clean, pure water.

Do You Know How Much Water Your Body Actually Holds?

Your body <u>holds</u> 'two thirds of an ounce of water per pound of body weight per day.**

<u>To calculate that amount:</u>
- Multiply your body weight times 0.66. That will tell you the number of *ounces* of water your body holds.
- Divide that figure by eight, assuming that there's eight ounces in the glass. The answer you get equals the number of *glasses* of water your body <u>holds</u>.
- The number of glasss you <u>*need*</u> <u>to drink</u> each day is <u>half</u> of that amount.

<u>Sample Calculation for a 150 lbs person:</u>
1. 150 lbs x 0.66 = 99 ounces of water held in the body.
2. 99 oz. / 8 oz. glass = 12.4 glasses of water <u>held</u> in the body.
3. 12.4 glasses of water <u>held</u> in the body / 2 = 6.2 glasses of water is the amount to drink each

---

If you've been drinking *more* **than that amount water**, and you're still thirsty, it is because you haven't had the <u>minerals</u> your body needs to integrate the water into the cellular fields. Remember, minerals provide the charge to move and exchange fluids through the cellular field. Does that make sense to you now? Can you begin to understand the importance of trace minerals?

If you've been drinking *less* **than the amount of water** shown by the formula you now know how much you need to increase your daily intake. And sorry, sodas and teas don't count.

To add appeal to water: use it cold, or use it hot. Put lots of ice in it or ice chips. Add a few drops of lemon or orange or lime, or whatever flavor you particularly enjoy. Sip at the water rather than chug-it. You'll find if you sip at it throughout the day, you can consume more than you think. Start sipping early in a day, but quit long about 7pm-ish so you get a good night's sleep.

Regarding Distilled Water

Recently, several patients have given histories of drinking distilled water as their everyday water source. Distilled water means the water doesn't contain any minerals. While there are some practitioners who advocate the daily use of distilled water, to this practitioner, that habit seems highly counterproductive to health. The Krebs cycle, your digestive process, requires a variety of minerals at *each* step.

Even with sources of minerals scattered around the globe, maintaining good levels of trace minerals is difficult, at best. Drinking distilled water - water leached of all minerals – requires the body to donate spare minerals you have lying around in order for your body to absorb water. This places you at an even greater risk of severe mineral deficiency! Since many disease conditions such as inflammation and pain are traced back to water and mineral deficiencies, drinking distilled water makes me shake my head. But, because this is such a hot topic in some circles, know that drinking a half-cup or so per day won't upset your apple cart too seriously. But the truth of it is, as a practicing physician, I personally don't recommend it.

Detoxifying - Even With
A *Therapeutic* Level Of Nutrients?

It can definitely happen. When your body has been without consistent levels of nutrients, many chemical processes haven't been completed, leaving inflammatory cellular debris lying around needing to be eliminated. Once you begin to take in nutrients, the body employs them as cleaning tools. With appropriate amounts of water to flush the cellular debris, your natural biochemistry will clean house! As debris is flushed out, it travels around in your circulatory system for a bit of time before being eliminated. During that time, it can be irritating to your tissues, so you may find yourself initially feeling tired or cranky, maybe impatient. This may or may not happen; but if it does, avoid biting someone's head off and drink another glass of water. This phase can last anywhere from 0 to 3 or 4 days, depending on how sick you were when you started. DRINK water! The sooner this is past the better. You look good with a smile on your face!

Cellular nutritional saturation is one of the three legs of health. It is vital for internal well-being, and its benefits are inestimable! You now know how critical the seven simple nutrients are for the human body.

Are you saturated?

Step Three

6

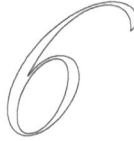

*Recognizing Sources of the Foods
That Cause The Body Pain*

"The doctor of the future will give no medicine but interest his patients in the care of the frame and in diet
and in the cause and prevention of disease."
~ *Thomas Jefferson*

Next Step: Calming Pain... Dare We Say *'Eliminate It?'*

During the first adjustments, as the structural components of the
body begin to regain stability and renewed nerve communication, as
solid nutrition and water begin to filter inward, it is amazing to witness the increase in nerve power. A patient's metabolic system
begins to percolate at a slightly higher plane. Your metabolic systems are your internal mechanisms that perform the automatic
tasks of everyday living. These systems are contained in the organs
that live in your abdomen and brain. Structural adjustments to the
low back, mid-back, shoulder girdle, neck, knees, skull and organs
allows all of those regions and their surrounding cellular parts to
become nutritionally refreshed and electrically empowered. The
whole body starts working better. Sometimes pain patterns continue on an intermittent and scattered basis with the body not yet

fully reconciled. When this happens, it's time to look closely at the diet.

In our first years of working with fibromyalgia, we encountered a variety of gastrointestinal dysfunctions instigated by the sacroiliac syndrome. In response, we developed a series of different nutritional treatment plans to improve metabolic condition. Though none of them were specifically designed to eliminate pain, we inadvertently discovered that a change of dairy sources (from animal to plant sources) could decrease joint and myofascial pain patterns *as much a 75% or more in a week's time!* It's a vast understatement to say our discovery is truly astonishing! But we witnessed this shift happen time and time again. I can understand if you think that's a pretty bold statement. We've had a number of patients who felt the same way. But those patterns have continued to be reproducible with other patients. Let me show you what they found.

On-going, Long – Standing, GastroIntestinal and Digestive Signs & Symptoms

Gastrointestinal and digestive conditions that are triggered, influenced and/or increased by the sacroiliac and spinal misalignments involved with Chronic Sacroiliac Syndrome includes: Shortness of breath, atrial fibrillation, colitis of a variety of types (including any involving the esophagus, stomach and small intestine or ileocecal valve, colon, or rectal valve), gastritis, esophageal blockages or spasms, Barrette's Esophagus, hiatal hernia, acid reflux symptoms of any and all types, bloating, difficulty with digestion, twisted or telescoping bowel, ileocecal valve (ICV) dysfunctions, appendicitis, constipation, diarrhea, bladder or urine infections and dysfunctions, caliber changes in stools, tendency to experience repeat bowel or urinary infections, gastric upsets, flu's or colds (more than once/year), decrease in taste bud sensitivity.

Natalie Baskin

Natalie Baskin wanted to add the benefits of *Frequency Specific Microcurrent* to the treatment plan she developed for herself since her diagnosis of Fibromyalgia. Due to the wonderful abilities to calm myofascial pain and numerous other conditions, *Frequency Specific Microcurrent* has become a mainstay of our treatment plans here at the Fibromyalgia Care Center of Oregon.

Natalie's diagnosis was Chronic Fibromyalgia secondary to Trauma, stemming from a back-breaking motor vehicle accident that occurred during her early twenties. Scarring of her muscle and fascia fibers had been a constant battle to overcome.

As discussed before, myofascial regions are the interfaces of the body where muscle and fascia come together, usually for strengthening and supportive purposes. Occurring at the interface where human muscle attaches to bone and/or to another muscle or sheath of fascia, these myofascial areas serve to 'bridge' and strengthen transitional areas of cellular change. Sometime these myofascial fibers become twisted or broken, becoming covered with scar material. Scarring restricts muscular motion, often causing whole body regions to become compromised and no longer fully workable or able to stretch.

While these facial sheaths can provide an internal path for fibrous scarring or a rapid spread of inflammation, new research shows they may also contain an important nerve network. Research is currently being conducted to map the nerve network of facial sheaths. The bottom line: the fascial sheath is an extremely important tissue to address if you ever want to improve chronic structural problems, as chronic, structural problems almost always create myofascial compromise.

Frequency Specific Microcurrent

Out of the last decade of the 20th century, one of the most exciting fields of research and discovery, providing enormous importance for the 21st century, is the field of microcurrent. Using micro- amperage to address cellular fields, hundreds of *specific* frequencies have been discovered throughout the human system. Turns out, each type of cell and/or cell part has been found to have its own *individual* frequency. Using the micro-amperage of these frequencies provides a specific direction to cellular action, provoking rapid cellular changes and cleansing. Cells start functioning.

One of the leading researchers in this field, Dr. Carol McMakin of Vancouver, Washington, has discovered and identified many of these cellular and metabolic frequencies. Grouping them together, in a therapeutic manner, she has created an ability for a practitioner to affect individual cellular fields, thereby directly addressing dysfunctions, irritations, secretions as well as numerous other conditions of a biologic nature... and addressing the problem in such a way as to get the cells to respond briskly. We have literally *witnessed* some quite remarkable repairs. Literally, visually *watching* physiologic changes occur. It is an amazing treatment technique!

While *Frequency Specific Microcurrent* has been found to be an effective treatment for pain control and metabolic stimulation, it has also been found to be effective for calming myofascial and degenerative issues throughout the body. Repairing the trauma of concussion and traumatic brain injury is another huge and important treatment arena for microcurrent usage. For those reasons, Frequency specific microcurrent has become an important part of our treatment protocols at the Fibromyalgia Care Center of the Oregon. Dr. McMakin's brilliant work has contributed an important body of knowledge - and treatment potential - for our fibromyalgia world (frequencyspecific.com).

Natalie Baskin

As Natalie and I began working together, my interest in fibromyalgia was just beginning to surface. The Governor's Task Force was in its early sessions, so the Fibromyalgia Care Center of Oregon hadn't yet been born (www.fibrocare.org/careenterhistory).

Natalie's microcurrent sessions allowed us time to delve more deeply into her history and pain patterns. Her story was similar to thousands of others I've heard during my nursing years. As a still developing young doctor, this was only the third or fourth time I'd really focused on fibromyalgia and myofascial patterns.

As she and I continued to work during her microcurrent treatment sessions, she frequently had to shift her body in order to be comfortable in her chair – a classic sign of Chronic Sacroiliac Syndrome. Despite good and timely chiropractic care, a good massage schedule and a conscientious nutritional approach, Natalie still had structural and organ difficulties she needed to manage each day, sometimes moment to moment. Not yet 50, she had broken six vertebrae in her lower back during a motor vehicle accident at the age of 22. That's the same nerve-filled area of the body where the largest of those fibrous fascial sheaths live. She had lived with myofascial restrictions for many years.

Chronic pain takes such a huge amount of energy to deal with on a daily basis, and Natalie and her husband had just adopted a young boy. They were thrilled to be new parents; she wanted to be available to participate in everything in her boy's life.

Scarring always means a shortening of the involved tissue, often pulling other tissue attached to the scar. If it happens to involve the myofascial tissue, hundreds of tiny pain receptors can be ignited with any and every motion. The debris from the inflammatory chemical changes that result from pain is very irritating to soft tissue, producing an additional inflammatory response, increasing the cellular debris. Inflammation adds to pain patterns, and another vicious circle is established.

Natalie's childhood as an active athlete, followed by a broken back and many years of compensation resulted in her specific version of Chronic Sacroiliac Syndrome. There was no wonder she experienced such a high degree of pain. The torque of her pelvis – with tightening, spiraled tractioning of its fibrous, myofascial nerve network – activated many of her trigger points, on a movement-by-movement basis.

As she stood, her head was slightly cocked to one side. Both her knees were slightly flexed. She spent so many years slumping with back fatigue that several levels of organ dysfunction developed: one at her gastrointestinal level, and another at the hormonal level (due to the degree of her cranial distortion).

Despite good progress from using *frequency specific microcurrent*, after about four weeks the pain and residual inflammation continued to be an issue Natalie had to endure on a daily basis. The worst of her difficulty was at her hands. The numbness and tingling at her hands and feet and upper arms was distracting to her life. Natalie began to accept it as accumulation of permanent scarring from her multiple sports injuries and accidents. Multilevel dysfunctional dual pathways of her spinal nerves caused ongoing gastrointestinal problems that she chalked up to the stress of being a grade school teacher in one of the major school systems in Oregon.

Her chiropractor decided to retire that year so she and I took the opportunity to reassess her entire care program.

Seeing The Problem In Front Of One's Eyes

Natalie disclosed to me the many problems she "learned to put up with." While the structural care she had received had been enormously helpful, we shifted our approach to her concerns. We paid specific attention to the z-axis – the spiral or torque component.

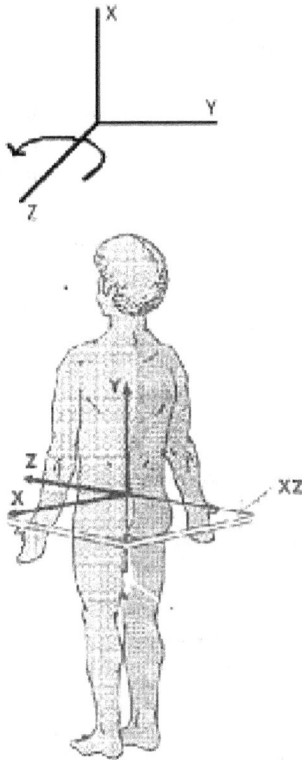

X, Y. Z axis

Active trigger points are *always* a sign that z-axis torque is engaged and a 'spiral' has been initiated. The torque tells you of the presence of the tilted pelvis of the Chronic Sacroiliac Syndrome the same way her inability to sit comfortably in a chair indicates the instability fostered by her sacral and pelvic tilt. The structural piece can't correct by itself.

Progressing Out Of Pain

Being a True Fibromyalgia of the Traumatic type, Natalie's Chronic Sacroiliac Syndromes stemmed from a torqued sacrum, setting up a spiraled spinal column, provoking trigger points both up and down her body. By correcting the positioning of her pelvis, tension was softened throughout her spine and her Trigger Points began to resolve. After that, her response was rapid. Within *six weeks*, she needed structural correction or adjusting only once every several weeks. By spring (we started in September), she was ATV-ing with her son. By the following winter, she was skiing!

Once we started taking the tension off of the z-axis, she was able to enjoy the loosening of her trigger points. Her response was rapid. Within *six* weeks, she needed structural correction or adjusting only once every several weeks. By spring (we started in September), she was ATV-ing with her son. By the following winter, she was skiing!

Inflammation & Pain

In the first weeks however, breaking Natalie's cycle of inflammation had to be addressed. When taming neuromusculoskeletal problems, tempering and containing the self-feeding patterns of inflammation becomes an immediate priority.

Two factors contribute to this easily escalated condition:
1) Inflammation is provoked through the cascade of histamine and prostaglandin release. It can be provoked by a.) irritating foods, chemicals/toxins, environmental allergens, or b.) the myofascial entanglements and scarring from structural misalignment patterns.
2) The second provocation of inflammatory episodes is through the accumulation of inflammatory debris. The presence of this

type of on-going problem is a sure sign of low vitamin D, imply-ing shortages of vitamin C, B-complex, and minerals. This is the point where you can see how and why microcurrent – com-bined with good nutritional saturation at the cellular level – provides such a good mechanism for acid-base neutralization and cellular rebuilding. Helps you see the need for the flushing with water too!

The microcurrent is the immediate calming and taming support; it interrupts the cycle of inflammation. Adding the nutritional satura-tion begins the cellular neutralizing of the body's cellular debris. Calming this inflammation can also be the slower side of the equa-tion.

It is not un-common for True Fibromyalgia patients to need four to six months for the initial stage of neutralization to become no-ticed in the muscles. In other words, while rare, there have been a few cases where it initially took 3 – 6 months to calm pain patterns. But microcurrent – and nutritional saturation – go right to the site of the problem: the individual cell. *Frequency Specific MicroCurrent* is the most effective treatment technique currently available for taming of the acute inflammatory conditions. Following with ade-quate cellular nutritional saturation to maintain the neutralization, Natalie began to thrive!

Getting a person out of pain and back into their lives means that <u>pain has to stop</u>, and all the parts need to be able to move so all systems work... smoothly.

For Natalie, by her sixth week of treatment, the nutritional satura-tion vastly improved her energy levels and staying power (meaning it improved the ability of her adjustment to hold). Her structural integrity caused her body to feel *stable*. Her gastrointestinal con-cerns improved, but still hadn't fully settled. The myofascial 'achy' component had not fully calmed down, either. I was used to my pa-tients becoming pain-free, but I was also still new in the development of working with fibromyalgia. Natalie wasn't improv-ing to the degree I was used to seeing in my patients. It was time for more investigation.

147

Apologies

With apologies to the animal dairy farmers of America, we need to talk about an elephant in the room: the amount of disease, discomfort and pain in our population that can be traced back to the consumption of this common animal-sourced food in our food supply.

Please note: we will not be discussing or suggesting vegetarianism. Instead, we will be talking about the damages and difficulties encountered from liquid meat (animal milk and products derived from animal milk) only, not solid animal meat. Most milk products are derived from corn or grain-fed animals. Corn and grain feed typically contain a mix of antibiotics and artificial hormones, over and above the ones ingested while eating the animal's solid meat, all of which are harmful to the human immune and digestive systems.

Food Causing Pain? *Food* Causing Pain!

Initially, our clinic didn't have the protocols and lessons about supplemental nutrition and food consumption that we do now. Natalie was among the first 'True' Fibro patients who taught me the extent to which our common foods *cause* (yes cause!), *exponenciate* and *magnify* pain patterns.

Working in the intensive care units as an RN, I was already well aware of the influence animal dairy proteins have on the production and thickening of mucus (with its nasty down-line effect on respiratory and gastrointestinal diseases). Specializing in fibromyalgia and other types of arthritis has since expanded my understanding as to just how pain-producing those proteins and contaminants are for both traumatic and chronic pain problems. In this book we focus on the chronic side of problems.

How Much Dairy Do You Eat?

Investigating a patient's dietary food consumption can be frustrating because as soon as I mention dairy products, people almost always say, "Oh I hardly drink any milk at all."

But, having studied dairy proteins for over 20+ years, I developed the ability to recognize evidence of the presence of certain proteins in a person's face and body. While they may not have been drinking actual *glasses* of milk, it is often obvious people were ingesting some amount of animal-fluids based products in their diet. We needed a way to determine that amount.

Designed to estimate a person's daily exposure to the many forms of dairy, The Food Survey showed us the truth in the observation of the havoc caused by the presence of those proteins. Patients are often astounded when they learn their degree of daily exposure to these foods. The Food Survey doesn't show the *amount of* dairy each person consumes, just the average number of daily exposures to some form of dairy product. It is not at all unusual to be able to see a link between the amount of diary consumed during a day and the amount of pain indicated by a person's pain drawing. Pain responses from consumption of any form of dairy seem to manifest anywhere on-the-average-of 30 seconds to three days after ingesting those 'not-meant-for-human' foods.

Semantics

In discussing my observations associated with the consumption of dairy products and the onset of pain patterns with other doctors and scientists in my profession, my peers would tell me "You can't say that animal milks cause pain. That's not good science." They would tell me, "What I *can* say is: *sometimes*, when *some* people consume animal milk, animal milk products or foods containing animal milk products, they *may* experience an IG-E mediated antibody response; and that *might* trigger a histaminic reaction leading to the production of prostaglandins, enzymes and/or neurotransmitters that *might* provoke pain receptors, *possibly l*eading to a muscular sensory pain sensation."

Over the years we have found that eating products containing animal fluids appears to provoke pain responses in the human structural system. Whether it is the proteins or the contaminants or a combination of both, I don't really care. What we watch is the **HUGE** change that occurs in a painful human body when dairy foods are sourced from plants rather than animals.

149

Hormonal Influence

It was the *hormonal* connection to dairy that initially caused Natalie and I to recognize the *pain* connection presented by dairy consumption.

Any time someone presents with a history of hormonal dysfunction, a chiropractor can find identifiable *structural* problems - usually in the cranium, pelvis and/or spine. These structural misalignment shifts can affect the expression, (production and/or secretion) of your major hormone and neuroendocrine glands: thalamus, hypothalamus and pituitary. Anatomically located within the middle of the skull, in a small bony pocket known as the crista galli, those little glands are affected by any unleveling of the uppermost crossbar at the jaw. Got a TMJ problem? You could have hormonal disturbances that may not be corrected by a pill. The tilt of your shoulder crossbar can compromise the distribution of the nerve flow from your cranial crossbar; and the torque of the pelvis affects how your adrenals work and respond to the hormones delivered from the thalamus, hypothalamus and pituitary. Your structural torque can really affect your overall hormonal output.

Whenever you have hormonal and neuro-endocrine disturbances, look first to the structure since your head houses those vital glands, the source of all your hormones. Minute cranial distortion of your cranial crossbar can prevent or compromise those glands from functioning normally. Correct that structural factor first and see what is left. If that doesn't correct the concern, then look to the diet.

Fifteen years of using the Food Survey shows us that an average person uses commercial dairy 3 – 8 times per day, with occasional bursts of more than 10 – 12 times per day.

Begin to notice the time when your pain patterns start to show up. How long ago did you eat? Was there any dairy in that meal? (Small amounts count.) You may have more control over your pain patterns than you're currently aware.

'IT'

To investigate food concerns in the 'sensitivity' or 'allergy' range, the first and best approach is through dietary elimination. Your frequency of bowel elimination determines the time needed to distinguish a food sensitivity or allergy. The slower the pattern of bowel elimination, the greater the potential to develop pain, inflammation and gastrointestinal disease. As my patients begin to eliminate animal fluids from their food intake, not only do their personal hormonal problems improve, they begin to report a large and rapid improvement in their pain patterns as well. Initially I credited chiropractic care for their improved pain sensitivity. But the repeated quick drops - some as much as <u>75% in a week's time</u> - couldn't *all* be put up to structural care. At least, not in THAT short amount of time: 7 days? There was something else going on here. Natalie was one of the first to help me define it.

At the end of her weeklong dairy challenge, Natalie's statement to me was, "I feel lighter, and my pain isn't *nearly* as bad either!"

This time I heard it. My ears picked up, as my head did a comical 90-degree whiplash turn. "What did you say?"

"I haven't needed nearly as much pain medication this week." she replied. Prior to that time I had only encouraged those patients with specific disease concerns (gastrointestinal, respiratory, cardiovascular, hormonal problems) to experience the diary challenge, not for <u>pain</u> concerns. Can those proteins and contaminants be that irritating to our tissue? Can they really be that influential on expression and production of pain? Could consumption of animal products be contributing to narcotic addiction problems?

Over the next year, I began to encourage everyone to experience the diary challenge. Even the people resistant to the news about dairy were willing to test the theory when they heard about the possible change of pain. Never once has a person, who has experienced this challenge, NOT had their pain patterns drop – not one of them! Now, 'it' all made sense to me.

'It' was an observation I had made during my last years as a bedside RN in the Intensive Care Units in one of our major west coast hospitals. There is a time, after each meal (assuming that patient is able to eat) when a patient either needs: 1) to have their throat or tracheotomy tube suctioned on almost a continual basis because of the amount of mucus suddenly being produced, or 2) will ask for a pain pill. It is such a routine component that you can almost clock it. I had done so daily, after each meal, for years!

The pattern was so universal throughout any given ICU or hospital population on any given day that I began to pay attention to the contents of food trays. Not all trays had meat, but ALL trays had some form of foods made from animal fluids: whether it was butter or yogurt or ice cream or cream soup or milk itself – some form of dairy was on each tray. I began to study dairy foods. The more I studied, the worse the information got.

Milk DOES NOT Appear To Do A Body Good

Proteins contained in the fluids of animals, some providing food for the human system, can, over time, cause the tissue it keeps alive to actually deteriorate into a dysfunctional state. Continue to consume animal products, maintaining a daily intake for decades in a lifetime and the dysfunction will accumulate into dysfunctional disease.

What Diseases?

We call these dysfunctions and diseases by the names of: Attention Deficit Disorder (plus a variety of other behavioral problems), arthritis, PAIN (*any* PAIN problem), asthma, allergies, Alzheimer's, anemia, bed wetting, bone disease, PAIN, bowel dysfunction, breast cancer, brucellosis, cholesterol and liver problems, chronic fatigue syndrome (CFS), colic, colds, congestive conditions, Crohn's disease, PAIN, Diabetes (both juvenile and adult), depression, dioxin poisoning, early maturity, fibroids, fibromyalgia, PAIN, endometriosis, hormonal imbalance, headaches, heartburn, infertility, kidney stones, lymphoma, lactose intolerance, leukemia, lungworms, amyotrophic lateral sclerosis (ALS), *any* autoimmune disease, PAIN, mucus problems, migraines, mood swings, multiple sclerosis (MS), nasal dysfunctions, obesity, osteoporosis, ovarian cysts, PAIN, prostate problems (both enlargement and cancerous), PAIN, rheumatoid arthritis, salmonella, sinus conditions, PAIN, skin conditions, stroke, PAIN, stomach aches, Sudden Infant Death Syndrome (SIDS), tuberculosis, the terrible two's, uterine cancer, colon cancer, PAIN, ovarian cancer, etc., etc., etc. (www.notmail.com; *Whitewash*, by J. Keon, MD; *The McDougall Plan; The McDougall Diet*, by John McDougall, MD; *Milk, the Deadly Poison*, by Robert A Cohen.)

WOW! <u>That</u>'s quite a list! How can one food affect so many different parts of the body in so many ways?

59 Hormones!

There is no such thing as "hormone-free" milk. In order to provide milk, an animal has to have just been pregnant. Even with the 'organic' dairies, there are still hormones in that milk that come from the animal itself! It's not possible to get milk from an animal that doesn't have hormones. Milk is the end result of a pregnancy... *rich* in hormones meant to feed a very large animal, and help them grow very quickly!

Today in America, each bite of anything containing commercial animal fluids has approximately 59 bovine and synthetic hormones in it. 59! *Fifty-nine*! About half of those (25 – 28 or so) are from the animal itself and *can't* be separated out of the milk. Those are the hormones designed to grow a 600 to 800 pound animal in 15 months! Could that have anything to do with our current obesity epidemic? Or the fact that our children are starting to grow breasts by the age of eight?

The other thirty some-odd hormones are determined by veterinary science to be needed to bring a cow to pregnancy and to provide the level of milk production demanded from each animal today. This equates to a total of fifty-nine hormones in each bite of anything made with or containing animal-sourced dairy. That boggles my brain! This is what we are feeding to our *babies*!

52 Antibiotics!

Added to the hormonal soup is another category of pharmaceuticals that can be every bit as dangerous and toxic to the human as the hormones. Each bite carries with it traces of fifty-two antibiotics. <u>52</u> antibiotics! These are considered by veterinary science as necessary for the growth, support of metabolism, and prevention and treatment of infections of this 600 – 800 pound animal. Fifty-two antibiotics. That almost chokes me! All in one animal. All at dosages for a LARGE animal. Leaving plenty of residues left over for any human consuming that food. Is there any wonder our citizens have such a heavy preponderance of gastrointestinal concerns? I know what just *one* antibiotic does to *my* system!

111

That means, every bite, of *any* type of dairy - or food containing dairy - put into your mouth carries with it traces of 111 hormones or antibiotics, all made of bovine or synthetic proteins that act as foreign substances to the human system! *One hundred and eleven!* (Remember that part about *"...IG-E mediated antibody response triggering...?"* Now multiply that response by one hundred and eleven.)

If it takes 10 pounds of milk to make a pound of cheese, doesn't that mean that every bite of cheese carries traces of 1,110 bovine or pharmaceutical compounds into a human body, with every bite? A pound of ice cream needs 12 pounds of milk; butter takes 21 pounds of milk per pound! Those are *dense* foods! Can you begin to imagine how and why we get so sick so often?

Can you begin to understand how the level of chemical disturbance occurring from 111 foreign particles (times however many bites of that dairy you eat on a daily basis) can be connected to the reality of any or all of those diseases developing?

But wait, there's more!

Today's Contents

Coming from a world today where so many foods are made and prepared for us by so many companies, restaurants and cultures, we tend to forget (ignore?) just how many products in our vast food universe are either made from cow's milk or contain bovine milk components. We Americans love creaminess!

Read the ingredients on labels of the processed foods you eat and see how often types of milk or milk proteins are contained in the ingredients. Look for words such as Casein, sodium caseinate, calcium caseinate, whey, curds, solids, albumin, MPC (Milk Protein Concentrate), and lactoalbumin. Notice how often they are listed in the top five, meaning there is actually a *measurable* amount of it present in the food. Take the food survey (be honest – you are only competing with yourself) to determine how addicted your individual system is to dairy.

Addicted?

Avoid taking offense to the word 'addiction' because that's what cow's milk actually does to a human: it addicts the consumer to the substance. That happens because casein – 85% of the protein from the bovine – morphs into a protein called caso-morphine. The purpose of that protein is to actually *addict* the calf to the mom's teat until the calf is able to eat solids. For the human, caso-morphine acts just like morphine in deadening us, slowing us down, fogging the brain, fatiguing the system and addicting humans to the product. If you consume animal products, you don't stand a chance of avoiding addiction to them. Every bite of dairy products provides another 'dose' of this narcotic, sustaining its suppressive actions. Given the daily intake of the average person, couldn't this caso-morphine factor be seen as a strong contributing factor for Chronic Fatigue Syndrome and depression problems in this country?

You may want to experience a dairy challenge to see how much the liquid animal proteins could be affecting your body and how much they could be promoting your pain patterns. John McDougall, MD, suggests 30% of the Asian community is sensitive to the dairy proteins, 50% of Caucasians have that difficulty and 70% of African Americans are affected adversely by these proteins. What could this daily consumption of liquid animal proteins, with all their toxins and contaminants, be doing to *your body?*

Have your ever experienced what it feels like to run your body *without* all those fats and proteins and pharmaceutical additives?

A Mini Tour

For those of you who feel this avoidance of animal milks is a simplistic approach, let's take a mini-tour of the average drop of milk in today's agricultural world:

> We're already talked about the 111 animal and pharmaceutical substances that any and every drop of cow's milk contains. In addition to the traces of those 111 foreign chemicals, you get to ingest the pesticide and herbicide residue from the grass, corn and grain the animal eats. Along with those substances, large (*huge*) numbers of bacteria and viruses (pathogens) are swept into your body through the consumption of animal dairy foods.

Some of those pathogens are known to survive pasteurization, allowing them to begin to multiply and re-grow as the milk sits, even when it is refrigerated. Ever wonder where that seemingly-out-of-nowhere morning sore throat comes from? Or that sudden onset of your irritable bowel problems? Or the sudden onset pain at the back of your arm, that was fine right up to dinner? Look back over your last day's food consumption, starting with your last meal. Chances are you'll remember that ice cream with Aunt Sally's pie or sour cream on your taco, or some other 'ordinary' dietary adventure.

And last but not least amidst the contents of an average animal's commercial milk molecule is the <u>blood</u>, accumulated from chronic sores on the teats of the animal; <u>pus</u> (also known as somatic cells) from those same chronic sores treated with antibiotics; and <u>feces</u>, a frequent result of those antibiotics and provoking inflammatory conditions. All of these particles are contained in those fluids that the FDA says is 'okay' for American consumption. These body emissions 'cannot be fully separated out' during milking sessions, so the FDA made it 'okay' by passing a law that says: 'the milk can be sold as long as it has no more than 750,000 pus cells/cc.' (The FDA report called them 'somatic' cells; a 'cc' is 1/3 of a teaspoon.) That's two hundred and ten million 'somatic' cells per teaspoon!

The type of serious or chronic disease that can accumulate from decades of daily consumption of animal fluids and their common contaminants depends on 1) the structural integrity of the human system, or the lack thereof, (affecting power supply to the parts); 2) the overlying genetic predisposition of your particular family strain, influenced by 3) the food history of the person involved.

Just the act of changing from animals' milk products to products made from plant milks (such as coconut milks, nut milks or rice milks) will improve your digestive and immune systems.

Dairy Challenge

One day it dawned on me that I had never experienced what my body felt like without those heavy fats and other components. Coming from the south, my family had a strong base of daily dairy consumption, which probably doubled on Sundays! That food had been part of my life, literally from day one onward. Would my body feel different? I had no idea of what kind of difference might occur.

My initial dairy challenge (I had to do three of them before I really 'got' it!) was in the early 80s, before all the wonderful plant-milk products began arriving on the market. Today, one can use the support of coconut and nut milks (containing no contaminants and provoking no disease) and avoid missing any of their favorite dairy flavors as they progress through this discovery week.

Side note: You notice I did not mention soy as a source for dairy products. Today, in America, there are no labeling laws commanding a food producer to be honest about the source of soybeans used for food preparation. One of our largest petroleum companies, responsible for much of the genetically-modified research, appears to have contaminated soy fields around the world, making it impossible to know which provide 'real' beans and which are genetically modified (GMO). It is being suggested that GMO soy may provoke kidney problems in humans. Until those labeling laws are in place (so you may truly know what you are buying), soy milk might be better kept as a secondary choice. As we go to press, this statement is also becoming true for trustworthy sources of corn.

Take that Food Survey. Find out how many times a day you reach for something from the diary kingdom. Relate your pain patterns with that intake. Does it happen right after a meal or several hours later? Is it still continuing to provoke pain the next day? Did it disrupt your sleep? An elimination challenge can give you some major insight as to how food relates to your body.

Elimination Week

The goal during my initial Elimination Week was to allow the dairy residues to clear from my body, to see if my body would feel different without that food. I also wanted to learn the effect that dairy had on me.

During the first day or two, the initial challenge was to remember not to 'go for' dairy foods. What else would I eat? What else WAS there to eat? My focus had been so strongly dairy-oriented, I found out that I had been living with blinders. There were HUNDREDS of other delicious foods to eat. My food choices actually tripled, quadrupled! This was a good thing.

Then came the part where I had to remember to read labels and ask for ingredients from the chef to avoid getting any dairy with my prepared foods. This turns out to be an important talent to develop, as so much dairy is hidden in cooking and it's easy to underestimate how much of whatever kind is present.

If you slip up, start your week over again. Yes, it makes <u>that much</u> of a difference. Each time you put those foods into your mouth, the body will stop eliminating and producing and accumulating mucus again. So my first 'week' actually took me a bit longer than seven days.

But it was worth it! My body DID feel different. It felt <u>SO</u> different! So <u>very</u> different! I was lighter, the fatigue was gone, I no longer felt I had to claw my way to consciousness after sleeping, or need to nap any time I sat down in a chair. I felt so much lighter. It felt almost as though I had springs under my feet. I was actually sleeping! Not just tossing and turning. Done before I became a doctor, my first dairy elimination was a crucial turning point in my understanding of the true influence food has in any given person's individualized health picture. It allowed me to realize I had much more control over promoting my health than I previously realized. It increased my <u>real</u> understanding of the power of foods and the need for adequate nutrition.

During the week I experienced a good mucus purge. Be prepared. Buy lots of Kleenex. Once you stop putting the mucus-producing proteins IN your body, your body can start digging OUT what has 'stacked up.' Don't worry about spitting out mucus or coughing it up or having it eliminated through other avenues like your bowels or urine. Keep your vitamin C intake strong and your coconut oil intake strong so you don't break down into a cold; but *let that stuff flow*. DON'T stop the progress.

Go completely without any forms of animal dairy for that full 7 – 10 days, depending on how often you move your bowels. Let your body feel the change before you have your 'challenge serving.'

On the 8th or 11th day, have one serving of whatever your food survey shows you use the most in any given day. Just one serving. Then watch what happens in your body over the next 30 seconds to 3 days. Watch the phlegm from your throat or runny nose, or the pain in one of your hips or back maybe, a return of a bit of fatigue maybe... observe whatever it provokes in *your* body.

That's what you have been putting up with. Learn about the influence of dairy on your disease conditions. Watch how often it provokes pain for you. Realize the degree to which you have been 'dosing' your pain and pain patterns… on a daily basis.

Other Foods That Cause Pain

Nightshades (potatoes, tomatoes, eggplant and peppers) and gluten (wheat) are two other categories of foods that provoke pain in the human, particularly in an already structurally misaligned person. The nightshades seem to have a proclivity for provoking pain at arthritic joints and inflamed regions. Gluten, a soluble fiber of grains, increases pain by slowing metabolism, contributing to cellular congestion and toxicity, increasing inflammatory conditions.

At the Fibromyalgia Care Center of Oregon, after what we've found with the degree of improvement achieved with milk source changes, the nightshade and gluten foods are seen as secondary contributors. Not to dismiss the havoc and annoyance nightshades and gluten can stir, but they appear to become exacerbated in the presence of animals milk.

Experience the shift of dairies before you scoff at this finding. In other words, after removal of the influence of the animal milk proteins, many of our patients discovered their bodies could tolerate and enjoy some of the nightshades and glutens. We suggest removing one food category at a time and see what is left. Ask yourself, what could right itself in *your* body if over 100 *foreign antigens were removed? Would your inflammation stop and/or start to clear?*

Setting Yourself Up For Success

When you focus on clearing food sensitivities with elimination diets, approach only one food group at a time. Avoid attempting to change the source of your dairy and banish gluten sources in the same time period, for example. That could set you up for failure. This book is intended to give you something that actually works. We intend for you to become a success. Give yourself time with each food group to be able to determine the true extent of its influence and cellular presence. Avoiding the food in its entirety for the necessary time period will give your body enough time to totally cleanse of that food. Allow a good six months to a year between food group changes. During the six months, keep your structural integrity intact and your nutritional bases strong all along the way.

Research further information about the connection of dairy with your specific concerns at www.notmilk.com.

Natalie

As she learned to substitute plant milk products for animal milk products, Natalie continued to improve structurally, metabolically and digestively. As she avoided dairy proteins and their contaminants, continued to get periodically adjusted and use the microcurrent occasionally, her pain patterns decreased to almost nothing. She learned how to substitute foods and sources for her dairy flavors, becoming very disciplined about keeping her body clean of malicious proteins.

She knows she is not 'healed.' Getting an adjustment every two to six weeks together with a *Frequency Specific Microcurrent* myofascial-pain-protocol treatment seems to be necessary to keep her myofascial scars at bay and "in their best" non-inflamed and pain-free shape. She maintains a strong nutritional base and watches the content of the foods she eats. But, between those times: there is just about nothing that she can't do these days!

Above And Beyond

Over the next several years, as she and I continued working together, Natalie would experience periodic flares of this or that joint. By that time though, it always seemed to be due to some sport-related type of stress, not toxic or metabolic stress. While the trigger points at her inside knees were among the last to go, they all ultimately faded away and her flares became less and less. Up until a short time ago, she hadn't had a flare in 6 years!

Ever Have One Of Those Lessons
So Thoroughly You Forget You Got It?

A few months after she retired, Natalie became bored enough to volunteer for – and was accepted by – the Oregon Search & Rescue

Team! In our state, this is a BIG deal. Oregon's forests contain thousands of trails and lumber roads; becoming disoriented and lost is easy to do in the best of conditions. Throw in some snow or a nasty period of rain and people can quickly get into trouble out there, without even trying. A searcher needs to be prepared for just about anything, in any terrain, in any weather. These volunteers are some of the most courageous heroes in our community!

Natalie went through the rigors of that training with strong, physical ease. That's how far she had come in conquering all of the scarring and toxicity compounding her version of the chronic sacro-iliac syndrome of her traumatic fibromyalgia. There was only once or twice she had to come in for extra treatment from bruising or falling down a hill.

About 3 years into her Search and Rescue duty – she had been out on some challenging rescues – she came in twice in one week, suddenly complaining of 'all that old aching again.' The barometer had been down, so maybe it was the cause. Her headache was explained away "because I haven't been drinking as much water as I should over the last couple of days." Her constipation tendency of the last week happened because, "I just haven't been exercising as usual this week." She said her sleep was upset due to the psychological anxiety of some recent family events. She told me her back pain was from a twist while climbing, and she figured she had just pulled a muscle.

Yeah, all that was possible. Until she came in a third time 3 days later, still voicing the same degree of symptoms and upset. That just wasn't Natalie at all. Something else was going on.

Knowing her diet had been fastidious for years, that she was very conscientious about checking food contents and avoiding certain categories of foods, off handedly I asked: "You couldn't have stumbled onto some dairy, could you?"

"No," she replied. "I'm pretty good at watching..." She stopped mid-sentence and turned to face me with that comical *'Oh-My-Gawd'* look of tragedy. "I've been eating a cup of yogurt each day this week!" She was irritated at herself; she knows better! She knows she doesn't even need to give up yogurt; but instead to get if from the wonderful coconut or nut sources available. She was somewhat irritated at herself, to say the least. Those personal self-sabotaging lapses can be pretty tough to swallow.

Which brings us to one of the understandings about dairy that I hear over and over from my fibromyalgia and arthritic patients. Once they get their body clean from those irritating proteins, they find that it doesn't take much exposure to animal proteins for the body to begin reverting into old pain patterns or increasing and thickening mucus production again. The pain and sinus symptoms seem to be the first symptom that people usually notice after a bite of something dairy. In other words, **it is not about the *amount* of that 'little bit,' it is the *presence* of the substance** that causes the problem. Little bits count.)

The next time you "just can't resist one little bite of cheese," ask yourself, "**Am I willing to be in pain over the next three days?**"

If the answer is *"No,"* then set the cheese aside and have some other wonderful (non-animal dairy) source of food. If the answer is *"Yes,"* enjoy the every little buttery molecule of each bite; then take note of when your first little twinge of discomfort occurs. It will most likely be somewhere between 30 seconds to 3 days after you take that bite, and will continue for somewhere between 3 and 5 days, until that bite of food finally exits your body through your bowels. Then, the next time a 'little' bit of dairy beckons, remember that twinge of discomfort and how soon it arrived. Is that how you want to treat yourself? Do you really *have time for the pain* and sinus congestions?

Once Natalie got over her chagrin at so smoothly dropping back into such a painful old habit, it took about a week for her to get back to her old self. With an old lesson newly relearned. Eating animal-sourced dairy products – even a little bit – can 1.) increase structural misalignment pain, 2.) increase mucus production, and 3.) increase inflammatory responses throughout the entire body.

7

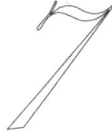

What It All Adds Up To

"Self-development is a higher duty than self-sacrifice."
~ *Elizabeth Cady Stanton, Cookeville, TN*

"It is achievable."
~ *Tarai Trent, 2011*

Take a step back and look at all of this from another point of view. Being subject to similar forces in our American lifestyle, many of us develop similar structural patterns as we go through life. The daily, hourly and minute-by-minute forces of gravity, vibrational compression accumulated from riding in vehicles and walking on concrete, provide tiny, compressive assaults on our structural system.

In the human body, nerves follow all the major bony paths. Each joint (along that bony path) houses *thousands* of microscopic proprioceptors, making-up those nerve-end organs that 1) monitor where we are in space, and 2) direct our structural ability to be in that space, guarding against missteps, possibly provoking misalignments. Misalignments interfere with the proprioceptors' ability to keep that joint - and its surrounding region - effective and strong.

As one neurosurgeon recently put it:

"Subluxations (misalignments) of vertebra occur in all parts of the spine and in all degrees. When the (subluxation) is so slight as to not affect the spinal cord, it will still produce disturbance in the spinal nerves passing out of their foramina (exit ports)." *James Wandersee, MD, 2012*

Each mechanical misalignment decreases nerve quickness and deftness, which in turn decreases the body's ability to structurally perform and behave in the way you would like. While misalignment patterns are similar in many people, each person has a unique pattern. Lifestyle choices (eating, drinking, exercising and/or engaging in specific activities) determine a person's exposure to certain types of daily assault, creating a uniquely acquired set of pelvic and sacroiliac misalignments. The unique set of misalignments can cause any combination of symptoms, such as low back pain, or neck pain, or headaches, or knee and foot problems, or shoulder problems, or gastrointestinal problems along with their accompanying symptoms (aches, pains, cramps, weakness, fatigue, etc.). Although structurally similar, each person's behaviors and choices are different, so each person experiences a different combination of misalignments and resulting symptoms.

Accumulated Cascade

The majority of Americans seem to glide through life with a minimal onset of structural problems. Any pain patterns they develop seem to be acquired more through periodic trauma than through accumulated missteps. A subset of people however, seem to be susceptible to developing a 'spiraled' tone to their accumulation of misalignment patterns. This spiraled tension can pull, buckle, torque or damage muscle and connective fibers to the extent of 1) dislodging the upper cross-bars of the body, thereby provoking changes throughout the upper body and spine while 2) igniting those nerve-end-organs known as trigger points. It can ultimately affect the tensional integrity your body needs to exert in order to carry itself about.

Disruption of this structural integrity can force a shift in your center of gravity, putting the sacrum off center changes the center of gravity to such a degree that a person can no longer depend on the pelvis to carry its weight. This is where the ability of the body to carry itself shifts from the pelvis to the shoulders... and starts involving the head to providing an assist in carrying the weight of the body. That expanding need for assistance starts to involve the muscles, causing overloads in localized small muscle fiber contractions... involving the trigger points. Trigger points are used to bear the weight of an abnormal posture. Your thoughts about 'increased neck tension' or 'shoulder tension' are REAL!'

By the time trigger points are involved, multiple regions of the body are already experiencing nerve confusion, already setting up the progression of any number of cascading regional or local joint, muscle and organ dysfunctions. The way the dysfunction is expressed depends greatly upon how a person habitually manages their body. This is where dietary and postural habits and exercise tendencies influence the outcome. Lifestyle habits can be an indicator of the type of symptoms that may develop, as well as where in the body the dysfunction occurs. The body begins misfiring in hundreds of ways. These are the people often diagnosed as having Fibromyalgia. It is this pattern of chronic sacroiliac dys-integrity pattern that is most often found on their initial examination.

Could 'Chronic Sacroiliac Syndrome' and 'Acquired Fibromyalgia' Be The Same Condition?

We have found a strong correlation between the case histories, physical examination findings, and symptoms of the Chronic Sacroiliac Syndrome of our fibromyalgia patients.

Over 25+ years, we've had numerous cases (each with their version of fibromyalgia symptomatology) clear up in the '14 to 90-day' period. Certainly not all cases clear up in that time frame, but length of time since diagnosis does not seem to be a trustworthy indicator of True fibromyalgia. The length of time spent struggling does not necessarily mean it will be a longer recovery. True fibro takes longer to respond, but we have not had any case where it does *not* respond. **Every patient, who stayed with the program, has responded to our three-step plan.**

We've had a small handful of people give-up on themselves due to the *slowness* of progress during their early days of recovery. Patients have also had family members give-up on them due to the slowness, causing the patients to give-up on themselves. Those who stayed the course improved and ultimately were able to get back into their lives to a far greater degree than they had previously achieved, needing less and less self-care along the way. Structural, metabolic and digestive stability IS a possibility without drugs.

How Do Chronic Sacroiliac Syndrome & Fibromyalgia Relate?

The structural pattern that appears to accompany the diagnosis of fibromyalgia is a progressive, mechanical, structural cascade occurring in response to the ordinary everyday structural and nutritional forces of life: normal gravity, the compressional vibration from riding in vehicles or walking on concrete, hitting your head on a cupboard, or stubbing your toe on the curb, or slipping off a step, or someone suddenly honking at you, arguing with your spouse, etc. Known initially (in the realm of chiropractic) as the Chronic Sacroiliac Syndrome, over a lifetime, this structural cascade appears to be able to progress in such a manner as to provoke the cellular and nerve-end-organ stress known as Active Trigger Points. Ignite enough of those nasty little points and a diagnosis of 'Fibromyalgia' can be made... a progressive, acquired accumulation of misalignments throughout the musculo-skeletal and neurological systems of the body provoking 1.) derangement of the structure, and 2.) dysfunction of the physiology and structural parts.

Nerves and muscles both depend on the skeletal structure for housing, protection, mobility and nutrition. Any shift in the structural integrity of the skeleton changes the ability of nerves and muscles to function, as well as changes *all* of their accompanying connective tissues and proprioceptive organs. Those structural changes, in turn, compromise the digestive and circulatory actions of the body.

What Do Chronic Sacroiliac Syndrome & Fibromyalgia Have In Common?

They exhibit the same types of structural and nutritional changes. Let's look at the structural component first.

Structural:

1) Both have a structural pattern that is similar in many humans, but unique to that person's lifestyle.

2) (Barring trauma), both are an acquired accumulation of misalignments that can occur in any and/or all regions of the body: from the pelvis to the spine, from the shoulder girdle, the skull, the elbows and hands, to the knees and feet – even throughout the abdominal organs. Over a prolonged period of time, nerve compromise from mechanical misalignment can change the action of nearby body parts. Organs dysfunction and tissues clog, as nutrients, oxygen and water are unable to get through to clean the areas. Disease builds. This happens as a result of interrupted and compromised nerve flow from acquired and accumulated structural misalignment patterns.

3) Both conditions are composed of a variety of diagnosable dysfunctions at multiple layers and regions of the body: pelvic, spinal, cranial, shoulder, extremity, neurologic, digestive, metabolic. Dysfunction can ebb and flow in severity during any given day or week.

4) Both can include any (or all) of the symptoms generated by the human skeleton when any one (or all) of the crossbars of the body becomes unleveled – individually or collectively. The five crossbars in the skeletal frame offer structural support to the tensegrity of the spine and its organs, as well as between the shoulder and pelvic crossbars. Additionally, the crossbars aid in structurally maintaining the normal integrity of the entire human body.

5) Misalignments of the pelvis and spine that occur in both fibromyalgia and chronic sacroiliac syndrome result in stretching or loosening the ligaments that hold body parts together. When ligaments are stretched, numerous pain receptors, located *within* the ligaments can be ignited, and thereby expand both direct pain patterns as well as referred pain patterns.

6) Each misalignment can and will be compounded by any or all environmental, emotional or physical insult or assault to the body, such as: smog, water pollution, emotional meltdown, stress, stubbing of toes, tripping, falling, bumping the head – not to mention the occasional incidental traumas of a motor vehicle

accident or divorce. Each insult or assault will take the pre-
existing *structural* condition and make it worse!

7) Both fibromyalgia and the chronic sacroiliac syndrome are affected by the positioning of the sacrum, the fulcrum of the body.
When the sacrum becomes misaligned, your skeleton can and
will shift, slowly following a spiraling pattern of misalignments:
reaching from the pelvis and spine, slowly spreading throughout the entire body. This multi-layered spiraled misalignment
pattern can (over time) cause a shift in the body's crossbars, affecting the body's center of gravity, requiring the body to
engage the help of nerve-end-organs called Trigger Points in
order to carry itself. Because of this connection, Chronic Sacroiliac Syndrome is considered (by some) to be the activating
mechanism of Trigger Points.

8) Misalignments and active trigger points make exercising an up-
hill battle! Muscles originate from – and attach to – bones. When
a skeletal part is out of alignment, you can exercise that muscle
all day long, but as soon as you stand up and walk away on that
misaligned part, the muscle will go right back into dysfunction
again! Muscles out of alignment can develop a tone but have difficulty *holding* a tone.

9) When they remain unaddressed structurally, both the chronic
sacroiliac syndrome *and* fibromyalgia conditions can be responsible for the development of degenerative joint disease and the
arthritic problems that cause many Americans so much pain.
Periodic adjustment of the structure lowers the tendency of arthritis and organ dysfunction to occur.

**10) Both conditions can be corrected, stabilized and restored
through the use of chiropractic care.**

Nutritional:

11) Both fibromyalgia and chronic sacroiliac syndrome have structural strength and stability when the body is adequately and
appropriately fueled, hydrated and exercised... and *don't* have
strength or stability *without the appropriate fuel.*

12) Both conditions are painfully compromised when the ligamentous system lacks a *consistent* saturation of the basic
fundamental nutrients required for everyday strength. In addition, both require adequate levels of water.

13) When the body is nutritionally deficient at the cellular level, both conditions lack an ability to fight the changes fostered by the misalignment and inflammatory triggers, becoming unable to prevent progression of either structural condition.

14) Nutritional deficiencies for either condition increases the sensitivity of the body to the environmental irritants and contaminants, making the body much more vulnerable to those influences. A malnourished body has a diminished ability to neutralize the inflammatory cascades provoked by irritants and contaminants. **Animal milks, in particular, have been found to provoke structural pain patterns.** A shift in the diet to using plant milks (with complete avoidance of animal sources) has been found to decrease fibromyalgia pain patterns by as much as 75% in a week's time!

How Are Chronic Sacroiliac Syndrome & Fibromyalgia Different?

The chronic sacroiliac syndrome may not be the *cause* of fibromyalgia, however the syndrome is *almost always present* in those diagnosed with fibromyalgia, either 'True' or 'Faux.'

The chronic sacroiliac syndrome appears to promote and be structurally responsible for the many symptoms associated with fibromyalgia.

The chronic sacroiliac syndrome does not include the myofascial-scarring components nor does it usually include the inflammatory components found with so many fibromyalgia patients.

Most people can correct the occasional problem of low back pain or plantar fasciitis or tennis elbow or headaches and go on with their lives. However, for too many other members of our society, the cascade becomes much worse, contracting and fibrosing connective and muscular tissue, provoking restrictions in mobility, creating organ dysfunction and serious pain issues, for years at a time!

Treating the condition as a disease over looks the need for correction of the structural nerve flow, preventing the muscular and metabolic problems from healing. Pharmaceutical drugs *quiet* the condition, but don't correct it. Merely quieting the conditions with drug use allows the structural compromises to continue to accumulate, progress and interfere. The conventional method of treating

169

the condition as a disease often neglects to <u>add</u> the basic foods and nutrients required for healing. You have seen how deficiency of nutrients is often a major cause of the symptoms.

Treatment Plans

How can you repair the body when even the best pharmaceutical medications haven't been able to temper the multiple problems that come under the diagnostic name of Fibromyalgia?

It's done by looking at the body as a <u>structural entity</u>, rather than a set of <u>*diseased* parts</u>, whereby a greater progress toward wellness can occur.

To correct the structure, we address the body by:

1) Correcting the body-wide structural misalignment patterns from head to toe, according to each body's individual needs.
2) Nourishing the cellular level of the body with the seven basic nutrients needed for the repair, function and growth of neurological, muscular, and skeletal tissues.
3) Discovering and removing any environmental factors that provoke structural or cellular havoc in that particular body.

These three steps seem almost too simple, yet using them as our mission guide, we have watched patient after patient calm their fibromyalgia pain patterns and ease their structural dysfunctions. While not all auxiliary diseases can be reversed, their progression has often been known to become tamed. People learn how to get back into their lives and STAY in their lives.

Step one is providing the care that creates structural stability and proper nerve function. Improved nerve function begins to immediately change the structural sacroiliac stance: starting from correcting the pelvis, strengthening and stabilizing the spinal position from the head to the toes. Correcting and empowering all the nerve flow out of the spine, gives every cell and every organ new power and energy.

Step two introduces the use of the nutritional POWER drink, with its concept of bathing the cells in adequate levels of the basic seven fundamental nutrients. All the structural and cellular systems start cleaning and throwing-out the trash. They can actually start pumping and breathing again. A person's sleep improves. The body can finally get some of those minerals and calcium that it has so desperately needed.

Step three identifies and removes havoc-makers from the internal environment. No longer needing to protect themselves from damage caused by the harmful substances, cells can actual become strong, supportive and pain free. It is not unusual to find liquid animal proteins to be a source of serious irritants, provoking numerous pain patterns as well as influencing a progression of the auxiliary disease problem known to accompany fibromyalgia. Changing the *source* of dairy proteins has created MAJOR, <u>dependable</u>, positive changes in pain patterns.

Conclusion

What if nutritional deficiencies (combined with nerve compromise from the structural misalignments) were keeping your body from being able to neutralize the irritating biochemical substances those same nutritional deficiencies promoted?

What if the presence of both misalignments and nutritional deficiencies resulted in your body becoming overwhelmingly inflamed?

What if your daily ingestion of various foods (containing irritating and compromising additives) actually caused you pain?

How do you *truly* know what type of disease or dysfunction you have until you address these three components of misalignment, nutritional deficiency and toxicity in your body?

By addressing those three steps, along with some cheerleading, of course, our patients are back into their lives, keeping pain patterns, depression and immobility 'in remission'!

Treat the basics!
Promote your natural structural stability!

Give your body what it needs to heal. Be consistent with self.
Remove your havoc-makers.
Get out of the way!

Let your body's magnificent innate abilities do the healing!

Epilogue

Techniques Used Here

The recoveries outlined in this book were facilitated through the use of Sacral Occipital Technique (SOT), a full-body chiropractic assessment, diagnosis and treatment system developed during the first half of the 20th century by Dr. Major Bertrand DeJanette, an Osteopathic and Chiropractic Physician. Dr. DeJarnette's research and documentation enabled him to develop a system of analysis, diagnosis and treatment that encompasses the entire body.

SOT works with the understanding that the body's integrity arises from one section of the body attaching to another section of the body, attaching to another section of the body, providing a balanced system that requires all of the parts to support the whole. The central pelvic changes influence the positioning and operation of shoulders, arms, hands, head, knees, feet and organs supporting the body's innate mechanisms with the biophysical ability to function. Structural, physiologic, metabolic and meningeal systems, all are addressed, righting the whole.

The body's ability to operate is affected by the positioning of the body while the positioning of the body affects its ability to operate.

Structure Determines Function
Function Determines Structure

Using leverage and the body's natural breathing rhythms, SOT corrects the partial-arc spiraling and the tilt of the pelvis is changed. That subtle change improves and empowers the spinal nerve connections, allowing both nervous systems of the body to perform as close to normal as is possible for that structure to achieve. Each correction takes you further back down the road you traveled to get to the point of dysfunction present when you and your doctor started.

You do NOT have to live in pain.

Directories to find practitioners of SOT in your area are available online:

> www.sorsi.com
> www.sotousa.com

Website resources for other products listed in this book:

> www.youngevity.com
> www.liquidlife.com

Addendum One

The Big Idea

by B.J. Palmer, DC

A slip on the snowy sidewalk in winter is a small thing. It happens to millions.

A fall from a ladder in the summer is a small thing. It also happens to millions.

The slip or fall produces a subluxation. A subluxation is a small thing.

This subluxation produces pressure on a nerve. That pressure is a small thing.

The pressure cuts off the flow of mental impulses. Then decreased flowing is a small thing.

Decreased flowing produces a diseased body and brain. That is a big thing to that man.

Multiply that sick man by 1,000, and you control the physical and mental welfare of the city.

Multiply that man by 5 million, and you shape the physical and mental destiny of a state.

Multiply that man by 130 million, and you forecast and can prophesy the physical and mental status of a nation.

So the slip or the fall, the subluxation, pressure, flow of mental images, and disease are big enough to control the thoughts and actions of a nation.

Now comes the man. And one man is a small thing.

This man is an adjustment. The adjustment is a small thing.

The adjustment replaces the subluxation. That is a small thing.

The adjusted subluxation releases pressure on nerves. That is a small thing.

The released pressure restores health to man. That is a big thing to that man.

Multiply that well manned by 1,000, and you step out the physical and mental welfare of the city.

Multiply that well manned by 1 million, and you increase the efficiency of the state.

Multiply that well manned by a hundred and 30 million, and you have produced a healthy, wealthy, and better race for posterity.

So the adjustment of the subluxation, to release pressure on nerves, to restore mental impulse flow, to restore health, is big enough to rebuild the thoughts and actions of the world.

The idea that knows the cause, they can correct the cause of disease, is one of the biggest ideas though. Without it, nations fall; with it, nations rise.

The idea is the biggest I know of.

Addendum Two - Food Survey

2008 © Created by Dr. Sunny Kierstyn RN, DC

How much water (water, not fluids) do you drink on a daily basis?

_____Glass(es)/quart(s)/half gallon/gallon(s)

What other fluids do you drink in a day's time?

Soda	_____ glass(es) or can(s) per day/week/month
Juice	_____ glass(es) per day/week/month
Coffee	_____ cup(s) per day/week/month - with sugar/milk/both
Tea (black/green)	_____ cup(s) per day/week/month - with sugar/milk/both
Tea (herb)	_____ cup(s) per day/week/month - with sugar/milk/both
Milk	_____ glass(es) per day/week/month

How often do you eat these foods?

Ice Cream	_____ servings per day/week/month
Cheese	_____ servings per day/week/month
Cottage Cheese	_____ servings per day/week/month
Butter	_____ servings per day/week/month
Yogurt	_____ servings per day/week/month
Buttermilk	_____ servings per day/week/month
Sour Cream	_____ servings per day/week/month
Cream cheese	_____ servings per day/week/month
Chocolate	_____ servings per day/week/month
Pancakes	_____ servings per day/week/month
Waffles	_____ servings per day/week/month
French Toast	_____ servings per day/week/month
Omelets	_____ servings per day/week/month
Mashed Potatoes	_____ servings per day/week/month
Baked Potatoes	_____ servings per day/week/month
Gravy	_____ servings per day/week/month
Buscuits	_____ servings per day/week/month
Croissants	_____ servings per day/week/month
Ranch Dressing	_____ servings per day/week/month
Blue Cheese Dressing	_____ servings per day/week/month
Creamy Soups	_____ servings per day/week/month
Bread	_____ servings per day/week/month
Donuts	_____ servings per day/week/month
Pizza	_____ servings per day/week/month
Hamburger	_____ servings per day/week/month
Cheeseburger	_____ servings per day/week/month
Chicken	_____ servings per day/week/month
Fish	_____ servings per day/week/month
Red Meat	_____ servings per day/week/month
NutraSweet/Equal	_____ servings per day/week/month

Score:

Score '1' for each time an item is eaten per week.
Score '.25' for each time an item is eaten per month.
Add them together to find the number of exposures you experience each day.

This form measures the number of times per day and per week that you expose yourself to liquid or food products from an animal. Count only those that fall into the realm of 'liquid' meat and Americans know or consider to be 'dairy.'

The number of times per week you are exposed to those foods often determine the amount of daily pain you experience.

References & Works Cited

For the purpose of simplicity, resources cited in more than one chapter are noted only once.

1. The immediate effect of individual manipulation techniques on their function measures in chronic obstructive area disease; DR knoll, JC Johnson, Robert Baer, Eric Schneider, osteopathic medicine and primary care 2009, 3:9 DOI: 10. 1186/1750 -- 4732 -3-9.
2. Assessment muscle shortening and standing posture and children with persistent asthma; Lopez, Prisco, Galvani, the owners, Jakob, at all, Department of physical therapy, school of medicine, University of Sou Paulo, Sao Paulo, Brazil, 11/2006
3. New guidelines from the BMJ on acute neck injury, Michael Friedman, PhD, January 2010
4. This from Dan Murphy; a collection of chiropractic statements by Dan Murphy, 2009
5. "Hey castles and how to deal with them," Dr. Kevin wall, to your health, January 2010
6. "Fibromyalgia, an Alternative View," Caroline McMakin, MA, DC, 2007
7. "Microcurrent treatment of myofascial pain in the head, neck, and face," Caroline McMakin, MA, DC, topics in clinical chiropractic, volume 5, issue one, 1998 pages 29 -- 34.
8. Treatment of resistant myofascial pain with microcurrent using specific microcurrent frequencies applied with graphite\vinyl gloves presented to the American backed society, December 11, 1997, Caroline McMakin, MA, DC.
9. "Fibromyalgia and the serotonin pathway," JH Juhl, DO, alternative medicine review, volume 3, number five, 1998, page 367 – 375.
10. "Emerging concepts in general biology of chronic pain: evidence of abnormal sensory processing in fibromyalgia," RM Bennett, M.D., neurobiology of chronic pain, volume 74 or April 1999, page 385 397.
11. Fibromyalgia, S. ChakraBarty, MD, R. Zooro, MD, American Family Physician, Vol 76, # 7, July 15 2007, 247-254.
12. "Internal Forces Sustained by the Vertebral Artery During Spinal Manipulative Therapy," BP Syons, DC; T.Leonard, W. Herzog, PhD, JMPT, Oct, 2002.
13. "Biomechanical Characterization (Fingerprinting) of Five Novel Methods of Cervical Spine Manipulaiton"; GN Kachud, DC; W. Herzog, PhD; JMPT, Vol 16, #9, Novc/Dec, l993.
14. "Central Hypersensitivity in Chronic Pain after whiplash injury," Curatolo, Petereen[Felix, Arendt[Neilsen, Giani, Zbinden,Radanov, Clinical Journal of Pain, o1 Dec 2001, 17 (4): 306-15
15. "Prognostic Factors Associated with Minimal Improvement Following Acute Whiplash-Associated Disorders," JA Duftn, Dc, JA Kopec, MD, HWong, BASc, PhD, JD Cassidy, HD, J Quon, DC, G. McIntosh, MSc, M Koehoorm, PhD, SPINE, Vol 31 #20, E759-E765
16. "Study Shows Even Small Difference In Leg Length Increases Disease Risk and Severity," WebMD, 12/2006, http://www.webmd.com/content/Article/129/117512 .htm?printing=true .
17. "A Review & MEdhodologic Critique of the LIteratrue Refuting Whiplash Syndrome," MD Freeman, DC, AC Croft, DC, AM Rossignol, DS Weaver, DC, M Reiser, Ph D, Spine Journal, l999, Jan 1;24(1):86-96.
18. Editorial: "Whiplash Injury, Biomechanical Experimentation, N. Yoganandan, P:HD, FA Pintar, PHD, M Kleinberger, PHd, Spine, Vol 24, # 1, pp. 83-85..
19. Class Notes: NeuroAnatomy; Head & Neck Anatomy, D. Neimi, DC, C. Anderson DC, Cleveland Chiropractic College, 1988.
20. Ogilvy JW, Braun J, Argyle V, Nelson L., Mead M., Ward K., "The search for scoliosis genes"; SPINE; 2006 March 15; 31 (six): 679 -- 81.
21. P. Wood, C. Ledbetter, M Glabus, L. Broadwell, J. Patterson 2nd; hippocampal metabolite abnormalities in fibromyalgia: correlation with clinical features. The Journal of pain, 2008: December 10, 1016 J. J. pain. 2008 07 003.
22. Unknown Author; "how inflammatory disease causes fatigue."; Society for science, 2009, February 17.
23. A worker at all; "rising prevalence of chronic low back pain"; archives of internal medicine, 2009; 169 (re-): 251 DOI:
24. Srinivas, G., Rao, MD, PHd; J. F. Gendreau, MD; JD Kangler, MD, ; "understanding the fibromyalgia syndrome."
25. D. McDonald's, G. L. Mosley, P. W. Hodges,; "why do some patients keep earning their back? Evidence of ongoing back muscle dysfunction during remission for recurrent back pain"; the Journal of pain 2000 and, DOI: 10.1016\J.pain.2008.002.
26. M. Olbermann, MD, K. Nebie, PhD, I see. Shuman, T. Holle, M.D., E. R. Gizewski, M.D., M. Mascjke, MD, P. J. Goadsby, MD, H. C. Diener, MD, Z. Katsarava, MD; changes to chronic decay; neurology, 2009; 73: the 978 -- 983.
27. D. E. Ingber,, M.D., PhD, "Mechanobiology and Diseases of Mechanotransduction" annals of medicine, 2003; 35 (8.), 564 – 77.

28. D.D. Nancel, PhD, E. Cremata, DC, J. Carlson, RN, M. Szlazak, "effect of unilateral spinal adjustment of Go-niometrically assessed cervical lateral flexion end range asymmetries in otherwise asymptomatic subjects); Journal of manipulative and physiological therapies, volume 12, number six, December 1989, 419-427.

29. R. M. Rosenzweig, PharmD, BCPS, T.M.Thomas, RPh, MBA, an update on fibromyalgia syndrome: the multimodal therapeutic approach, American Journal of lifestyle medicine, February 24, 2009, DOI: 10, 1177\1559827609331557.

30. H.vanPraag, "exercise in the brain: something to chew on, trends in neuroscience is, volume 32, number 5, 283-290.

31. Antithrombotic Trialists (ATT) Collaboration, "aspirin in the primary and secondary prevention of vascular disease: collaborative meta-analysis of individual purpose data from randomized trials"; man sets, volume 373, May 30, 2009, 1849 -- 1860.

32. Fibromyalgia treatise, Dr. Adam Locke, DC, 2009

33. P. Belon, J. Cumps, M.Ennis, P>F> Mannaioni, M. Roberfroid, J. Sainte-Laudy, FAC, Wiegant, "you mean patients modulate cell activation," inflammation research, volume 53, number 5/April, 2004, 181188.

34. I.Azanon, P. Hggard, I "some sensory processing and body representation," science digest, 45 (2009) 1078 - - 10 84.

35. J. Legaye, G. Duval-Beaupere, "gravitational forces and sagittal shape of the spine.," international orthopedics, (S I COT) (2009) 32:809 – 816

36. D.R. Seaman, DC, MS., C.Cleveland III DC, "spinal pain syndromes: no CSF did, neuropathic, and psychologic mechanisms," Journal of manipulative and physiological therapeutics, volume 22, number seven, September 99, 458 -- 472.

37. L.Barclay, MD, " obesity paradox probed in new review," CME.medscape.com, 6/5/2009,http://cme.medscape.com/viewarticle/703966_print.

38. JR Taylor, P. Finch, "acute injury of the neck: anatomical and pathological basis of pain." Ann Acad Med Songapore, 1993 March; 22 (two): 187 – 92.

39. JD Drake, DP Callaghan, "intervertebral nerve for RAM and a determination to two types of repetitive combined loading" clinical biomechanics, 2009 January; 24 (one): 1-6.

40. AJ Bartsch, LG Gilbertson, V. Prakash, DR MOrr, JF Wiechel, "minor crashes and whiplash in the United States," Annu Proc Assoc Adv Autojot md, 2008 October; 52:117 – 28.

41. DP Swiercinsky, PhD, "mild traumatic brain injury versus posttraumatic stress disorder." Reviewer's letter,http://www.brainsource.come/mtbivs.htm

42. R. Pfeiffer,L. Pfeiffer, mild traumatic brain injury and postconcussion syndrome, 2007, course notes .

43. F.R. Carrick, PhD, E. Oggero, PhD, G. Pagnacco, PhD, ; posh graphic changes associated with music learning; Journal of alternative and complementary medicine; volume 13, number five, 2007, PP. 519 -- 526.

44. FR Carrick, DC PhD, changes in brain function after manipulation of the spine, Journal of manipulative and physiological therapeutics; volume 20, number eight, October, 1977 529 – 545.

45. CSM Bexander, R. Mellor, P:W Hodges, effective case direction on muscle activity during cervical rotation, Journal of an experimental brain research, 2005 December; 167 (three): 422 – 32.

46. F. Carrick, DC, PhD, the treatment of cervical dystonia bimetal manipulation of the cervical spine: a study of brain hemisphere at the, patient attributes, and dystonia characteristics.

47. RG Heath, brain function in epilepsy: midbrain, medullary, and cerebellar interaction with the rostral forebrain; Journal of neurology, neurosurgery and psychiatry, 1976, 39, 1037 – 1051.

48. D.E. Ingber, integrity one. Cell structure and hierarchical systems biology, Journal of cell science, 116, 1157 -- 1173 2003.

49. DE Ingber, integrity to. Structural works influenced cellular information processing networks, Journal of cell science, 116, 1397 -- 1408, 2003.

50. Y.Drory, "sexual activity and cardiovascular risk.," European heart Journal supplements, (2002) for (supplement H.), age 13 -- H. 18.

51. doctors of chiropractic serving as primary care physicians lead to better clinical and cost outcomes, Journal of manipulative and physiological therapeutics, therapeutics, June 2004.

52. studies document benefits of chiropractic care; a health insurance plan with the chiropractic benefit at lower costs than a plan without it, archives of internal medicine, October 2004.

53. Studies document benefits of chiropractic care: to be most effective, chiropractic care should be tried immediately after an injury, Journal of occupational and environmental medicine, January 2004.

54. Hu, FB, Obesity & mortality: Watch your waist, not your weight. Archives of internal medicine, 2007, May 14: 167:875 – 6.

55. Welty, FK,Lee, KS,Lew, NS,Zhou, JR, "effective soy nuts on blood pressure and lipid levels in hypertensive, hypertensive, in normotensive postmenopausal women". Archives of internal medicine, 2007, 167:1060 – 1067.

56. L.Barclay, MD, guidelines issued for management will: Medscape medical news: October 2, 2007; HDTV://www.Medscape.com/viewarticle/563639?src=mp.

57. JE Bialosky, PT, S George, PT, MD Bishop, Pt, "spinal manipulative therapy works: we. Why ask why?," Journal of orthopedic and sports physical therapy, volume 30 number six, June 2008, 293.

58. JA Zware, MD, G.Dyb, MD, K.Hagen, MD, S. Svebak, PHD, IJ Stovner,MD J. Holmen, Md, "analgesic overuse among subjects with headache, neck, and low back pain; neurology, May, 2004 1540 – 1544.

59. B. McKechnie, DC, DACAN, "cervical spine lytic myelopathy: useful clinical signs, dynamic chiropractic, January 29, 1993, volume 11, volume 11, issue 03.

60. K. Tracy, MD, "test discover a direct route from the brain to the immune system; Feinstein Institute for medical research, 2007,
http://hy143w.bay143.mail.live.com/mail/:PrintShell.aspx?type=message&cpids=c0c878cc:

61. C.Fernandez-de-las-Penas, PT., M.Perez-de-Heredia,OT, M. Brea-Rivero, OT, JCMiangolarra-Page, MD, "media effects on pressure pain threshold follow a single cervical spine manipulation in healthy subjects, Journal of orthopedic and sports physical therapy, volume 37, number six, June 2007, 325 – 329.

62. MJ Bolland, PA Barber, RN Dlught;y, B Mason, A. Horne, R. Ames, GD GANble, a Grey, IR Reid, "that's events in healthy older women receiving calcium supplementation: randomized controlled trial," British medical Journal, DOI: 10.1136/bmj.39440.525752.BE (published January 15, 2008).

63. "Sexual function in men and women after anterior surgery for chronic low back pain." 2006 May; 15 (five): 677 -- 82. Epub 2005, Sept 7.

64. SM Rubinstein, DF, DL KNol, PhD, C. Leboeuf-Yde, DC, MW vanTulder, PHD, "the nine adverse events following chiropractic care pain associated with worse short-term outcomes, but not worse outcomes at three months". Spine, volume 33, number 25, PP E950 -- E956.

65. Maigne, R., "Thoracolumbar Junction syndrome, a source of diagnostic errors, orthopedi c – thoracolumbar junction syndrome; http://www.maitrise-orthop.com/corpusmaitri/orthopaedic/mo70_maigne_thoracolumbar/.

66. Guez, M., Hildingsson, C., Nasic, S., Toolnen, G., Acta Orthop. 2006, Feb;77(1);132-7.

67. Groch, J., "exercise me that causes nor pretense knee osteoarthritis.";
http://www.medpagetoday.com/rheumatology/Arthritis/dh/4971.

68. Okifuji A., Truk, DC, Sex hormones in pain and regularly menstruating women with fibromyalgia syndrome, the Journal of pain, November 2006; volume 7, issue 11, PP. 851 – 859.

69. Angst F., et al, interdisciplinary rehabilitation in fibromyalgia and chronic back pain: a prospective out-comes study. The Journal of pain and, November 2006: volume 7, issue 11, PT. 807 – 815.

70. Editorial: N. Gevitz, PhD, "Center or periphery? The future of osteopathic principles and practices, , Journal of American osteopathic Association, volume 106, number three, March 2006, 121 – 129.

71. L.Tobias, "loosen up,". Times, September 2005, 23 – 20.

72. G.Kolata, NYTimes, "back pain sufferers to contest spinal procedure.," register guard, August 28, 2005.

73. S. Cuthbert, DC, "the importance of proprioceptive testing chiropractic, dynamic chiropractic, September 13, 2004, 8 – 10.

74. A. DeSienna, DC, "drug markup," public letter:
http://by106fdbay106hotmail.msn.com/cgi=bin/getmsg?msg=GA11584F-241E45CF-9B 5.17.2005.

75. "Lyme disease: diagnosis's," CDC is a perfect airborne infectious diseases,
http://www.cdc.gov/ncidod/dvbid/lyme/diagnosis.htm.

76. "Lyme disease: introduction," CDC division of vector borne infectious diseases,
http://www.cdc.gov/ncidod/dvbid/lyme/index/htm.

77. A.Apkarian, "chronic pain may shrink brain.," the Journal of neuroscience, November 23, 2004.

78. C. Gorman, A. :Park, "the fires within: inflammation is the body's first defense against infection, but when it goes awry, it can lead to heart attacks, colon cancer, Alzheimer's and a host of other diseases, Time maga-zine, February 23, 2004.

79. MM Panjabi, PjD, SIto, MD, AM Pearson, BA, PC Ivancic, MPhil, "injury mechanisms of the cervical vertebral test simulated whiplash," Spine, volume 29, number 11, PP 1217 -- 1225, 2004.

80. A. Sapega, MD, "Arthur fibrosis (Stephanie syndrome).," the knee and shoulder centers,
http://www.kneeandshoulder.md/print/print.arthro.html.

81. FM Lomoschitz, CC Blackmore, SK MIrza, FA Marin, "cervical spine injuries in patients 65 years old type, and stability of injuries." American Journal of rheumatology: 178, March 2002 573 – 577.

82. NJHolland, GM Weiner, "recent developments in bells palsy," British medical Journal, 2004; 329, 553557 (4 September).

83. Chiropractic Research Review: "diagnostic imaging: sacral liquidity: a useful gauge of normal lumbar pelvic silent spinal alignment.": fall 2004, April.

84. S.Kelleher, D Wilson, "the hidden be business behind your doctor diagnosis," the Seattle Times, Monday, June 27, 2005, http://by.106fd.bay.106.hotmail.msn.com/cgi[gin/getmsg?msg=?EBFIE8-3209-40CC-969...6/28/2005.

85. J. Kluger, "Blowing a gasket: more than 65 million Americans suffer high blood pressure, and that number is sure to rise. What you can do to control your" Time magazine, December 6, 2004.

86. JW Chung, Rohrback, WD McCall, JR, "effect of increased sympathetic activity on electrical activity from myofascial pain areas." American Journal of physical medicine and rehabilitation, 2004, November; 83 (11): 842-850.

87. J. Kurnik, DC, "breath in this sacroiliac joint," dynamic chiropractic/DC diagnosis and treatment November 18, 2004.

88. G. Null, PhD, C Dean, MD, ND, M. Feldman, MD< D. Rasio, MD, D. Smith, PhD, "Death by medicine", life extension, 2005.
89. B. Lipton, PhD, "insight into cellular consciousness closed quotes, Bridges, 2001; volume 12 (1): 5 pp. 425 – 462.
90. B. Lipton, PhD, "The evolving science of Chiropractic Philosophy, Part One," sees chiropractic, that is 88:60.
91. RM Bennett, MD," fibromyalgia and the disabilities dilemma: new concepts in understanding a complex multi-to pick me multidimensional pain syndrome," arthritis and rheumatism, volume 39: PP. 1627 -- 1634, 1996.
92. JW Potter, "Social Security: the role of the physician," fmaware.org/patient/disabilitypotterphysicianhtm.html.
93. J. Mercola, ND, "the truth about chiropractic, and how it is understood." http://www.merola.com/2004/feb/4/truth_chiropracatiac.htm
94. M. Descafreaux, JS Blouin, M Drolet, et al, "the figure she prevented spinal manipulation for chronic low back pain and related disabilities: a preliminary study," Journal of manipulative and physiological thera-peutics, October 2004; 27 (A.): 509 -- 514.
95. J. Mercola, ND, "chiropractic validates by medical research, www.mercola/2004/jun/30/chiropractic_validated.htm
96. J. Mercola, ND, "Beyond Bad Backs: what chiropractic is and how it can help you." http://www.mercola.com/2004/now/12/beyond_bad_backs.htm
97. JJ Collins, DC, "referring your patients to a chiropractor: a guide for MDs & DOs, hometown.aol.com/spabkchiro/myhomepage/business.html.
98. C. Kent, DC et al, "Chiropractic Influence On Oxidative Stress And DNA Repair," Journal of vertebral sublux-ation research, www.jvsr.com.
99. JHBland, SMCooper, "osteoarthritis: a review of cell biology involved in evidence for reversibility. Man-agement rationale it is related to know Genesis and pathophysiology" Seminars and Arthritis and Rheumatism , volume 14, number two, November, 1984.
100. "Manipulation in ASP care they take care loan for LBP," chiropractic research review, volume 8, number one, Winter 2005.
101. "The enemy within," the Journal of the American Medical Association, November 2003.
102. L. Feinberg, DC, "NMT: your pathway to wellness." NMT: The Feinberg Technique, 2003.
103. G. Crofton, " 'C' word raises red flags: national fibromyalgia Association founder says he's heard about cures before.," Lake Tahoe Daily Tribune, http://www.tahoedailytribune.com/article/2005418zmred104180010/-1/NEWS.
104. J McAviney, MS, D Schulz, BSc, DE Harrison, DC, B Holland, PhD, "determining the relationship between cervical lordosis **and** neck complaints," Journal of Manipulative and Physiological Therapeutics, March April 2005, volume 28, number 3.
105. L. Glennon, "How to Have a Healthy Doctor Patient Relationship," Ladies Home Journal Life, August 2004, 142 – 150.
106. S Simon, Md, RPh,"chronic pain management Paradigm: Time for change? Medscape, May 2004.
107. RW Goen, MD," the new nutrition and doubting doctors," the new nutrition. I'm, 12, 2001, http://www.studentsforlife.net/NewNutritionParadigm.html
108. R. LEchnyr, PhD, DSW, HHHoines, MD, "taxonomy of pain patient behavior," practical pain management, September October 2002, 18 – 25.
109. R. Lechnyr, PhD, "Psychological "Dimension of Pain Management, "Practical Pain Management, July/August, 2003, 10 – 18.
110. DG Williams, ND, "The Clock is Ticking," Alternative for the Health-Conscious Individual, volume 10, number 13, July, 2004 97 – 104.
111. J Whitaker, MD, "indicating illness," Health and Healing, volume 14, number six, June 2004, 1 to 8.
112. TT Davis, MD, RB Delamarter, MD, P Sra, MPH, TB Goldstein, MD, "the IDE T procedure for chronic low back pain," Spine: volume 29 (7) 2004 Pp 752 – 756.
113. "11 essential questions: provided by the Institute for safe medication practices." National Fibromyalgia Association, Online, volume 4, number 4, April 16, 2004.
114. TP Huttl, MW Wichmann, B Reichart, TKG Eiger, FW Shildgert, G Mey, "Lacroscopic Diaphragmatic plica-tion: long-term results of a novel surgical technique for postoperative phrenic nerve palsy," *Surgical Endoscopy*," March 2004.
115. DG Williams, ND, "magnetically attractive healing," Alternative for the Health-Conscious Individual, volume 10, number nine, March, 2004, 65 – 72.
116. "Chiropractic and its use in treating low back pain," National Center for Complementary and Alternative Medicine, Research Report, http://www.nccam.nih.gov/health/chiropractic/index.htm
117. A. McLellan, "safe and sound," Health Sciences, November 2003, p. 2-13.
118. J Whitaker, MD, "How to Stay Out of the Hospital," Health and Healing, November 2003, volume 13, number 11.
119. D. Uslan, MA, MBA, LMHC, "Reconstructing Your Life," January 2004.
120. B. West, ND, "The poly pill cure for heart attack and stroke," *Health Alert*, issue 10, October.

121. A. Robeneiks, "Hospital Patient Safety Effort Launched to Reduce Errors, Save Lives," Amed news.com, http://www.ama-assn.org/amednews/2005/01/03/prsb0103.htm.
122. JA Cambron, M Rudavalli, M McGFregor, J Jedricks, M Keenum, AJ Ghanayem, AGPatwardhan, SE Furner, "Amount of healthcare and self-care following a randomized clinical trial Comparing Flexion Distraction with Exercise Program for Chronic Low Back Pain," *Chiropractic and Osteopathy*, 2006, 14:19.
123. MR Gudavalli, JA Cambron, M McGregor, J Jedlicka, M Keenum, AJ Ghanayem, AG Patwardhan, "A Random-ized Clinical Trial in Subgroup Analysis to Compare Flexion Distraction with Active Exercise for Chronic Low Back Pain," *European Spine Journal*, 2006, Vol. 15:1070 – 1080.
124. Who Guidelines on Basic Training in Safety in Chiropractic, World Health Organization, Geneva, 2005.
125. AJ Terret, DC, "Concepts In Acute Basilar Complications Following Spinal Manipulation," *NCMIC*, 2001.
126. AJ Terret, DC, "Vertebrobasilar Stroke Following Manipulation," *NCMIC*, 1996.
127. G Plaugher, J Alcantara, RW Dobie, "This Sacral Fracture before Chiropractic Adjustment," *Journal of Ma-nipulative and Physiological Therapeautics*, September 96, vol. 19, issue 8.
128. "M.D.'s Cervical Manipulation Causes Woman Stroke," throw.com, December 20, 1991, volume 09, issue 26, http://www.chiroweb.com/archives/09/26/04.html
129. R Dziewas, et al, "Cervical Artery Dissection - Clinical Features, Risk Factors, Therapy and Outcome In 126 Patients," *Journal of Neurology*, volume 250, issue 10, October 2003, 1179 – 84.
130. DA Rivett, et al, "Effect of Pre-Manipulative Tests on Vertebral Artery and Internal Carotid Artery Blood Flow: A Pilot Study," Journal of manipulative and physiological therapeutics, 01614754, July/August 99, volume 22, issue 6.
131. BP Symons, DC, T Leonard, W Herzod, PhD, "Internal forces sustained by the vertebral artery During Spinal Manipulative Therapy," *Journal of Manipulative and Physiological Therapeutics*, volume 25, number 8, p. 504 – 510.
132. PB Licht, MD, PHD, HW Christensen, DC, MD, PF Hoilund-Carlsen, MdDMSc, "Is Cervical Spinal Manipula-tion Dangerous?," *JMPT*, volume 26, number 1, p. 48 – 52.
133. H Theil, G Rix, "Is It Time to Stop Functional Pre- Manipulation Testing of the Cervical Spine," *Manual Therapy*, May 2005; vol 10, p. 154 – 8.
134. E Ernst, "Manipulation of the Spine: A Systematic Review of Case Reports of Serious Adverse Events, 1995 - 2001," *Medical Journal of Australia*, April 2002, volume 176, issue 8, p. 376 – 80.
135. ELHurwitz, PDAker, AHADams, AWC Meeker, etal, "Manipulation and Mobilization of the Cervical Spine: A Systematic Review of the Literature," Spine, volume 21, 1996, 1746 – 59.
136. WSmith, etal, "Spinal Manipulation Therapy Is an Independent Risk Factor Vertebral Artery Dissection.," Neurology, volume 60, 2003, 1424 – 8.
137. BPSymones, MSx, DC, MWestaway, BSc, PT, "Virchow's Triad Spinal Manipulative Therapy of the Cervical Spine," Journal of the Canadian chiropractic Association, 2001:45 (four), 225 – 231.
138. PBLIcht, HW Christensen, etal, "vertebral artery flow in spinal manipulation That: a randomized That, controlled and Observer Blinded Study.," Journal of manipulative and physiological therapeutics, March 1998, volume 21, issue three. P1 41.
139. MJHaynes, BASc, "vertebral arteries and cervical Movement:Doppler Ultrasound Velocimetry for Screening before Manipulation," Journal of manipulative and physiological therapeutics, volume 25, number nine, 556 – 567.
140. MHaneline, DC, FICR, "chiropractic manipulation in the presence of acute cervical Vertebral Disc Herni-ation," dynamic chiropractic, December 1, 1999, volume 17, issue 25 http://www.chiroweb/com/archives/17/25/07.html.
141. JP Ladermann, "Cerebrovascular Accidents Related to Chiropractic Care That: for the Considerations.," European Journal of Chiropractic , 38, 1990.
142. AGTerrett, "Nice Use of the Literature Medical Offers in Discussing Spinal Manipulative Therapy Injury.," Journal of manipulative and physiological therapeutics, volume 18, issue four, 1995, 23-210.
143. PLynch, "Since the Neurological Injury Following Neck Manipulation.," Irish medical Journal, 1998, volume 91, page 130.
144. TCMichaud, "Uneventful Upper Cervical Manipulation in the Presence of the Damaged Vertebral Artery," Journal of manipulative and physiological therapeutics, September 2002 472 -483.
145. RKitchen, "nonunion (Type II).Doit Fracture: A Case Report of a Motor Vehicle Accident.," the Journal of the Canadian chiropractic Association, volume 30, number four, December 1987, 189 – 93.
146. JDorak:, "Inappropriate Indications and Contraindications for Manual Therapy," Journal of manual medi-cine That: volume 6, number three, 1989, 85 – 8.
147. AWFuhr, DC, JMMenke, MA, DC, "Activator Methods Chiropractic Technique.," EB SCO publishing, 2002.
148. "Most Common Causes of Chiropractic Malpractice Lawsuits.," Journal of manipulative and physiological therapeutics, of 161-4754, January 1997, volume 20, issue 1.
149. MIGattrman, MA, DC, "Standards of Practice Relative to Complications and Contraindications to Spinal Manipulative Therapy," The Journal of the CCA, volume 35, number four, December 1991 232 – 236.
150. PTehan, P Gibbons, "spinal manipulation That: indications, risks and benefits That.," Journal of bodywork and movement therapies That, volume 5, number two, April 2001, 110 – 119.

183

151. SHaldeman, DC, PhD, MD, SM Rubinstein, DC, "The Precipitation or Aggravation of Musculoskeletal Pain in Patients Receiving Spinal Manipulative Therapy," Journal of manipulative and physiological therapies That, volume 16, number one, January 1993, 47 – 50.

152. PCote, "Site Posture Manipulation and Lumbar Spine Disc Herniation: Where Is the Evidence Say?" 1998 International Conference of Spinal Manipulation: July 16 19, 1998, Vancouver, Canada.

153. RAPistalese, BSc, "risk assessment of neurological and/or Vertebrobasilar Complications in the PS3 Chiropractic Patient," the Journal of vertebral subluxation, June 1996, 77 – 86.

154. MTHaneline,DC, GLawkovich, DC, "critique of the Canadian stroke consortiums spontaneous versus traumatic arterial dissection Study.," Journal of the American chiropractic Association, may 2004 18 – 22.

155. PJ Pronovost, MD, PhD, et al, " senior executive Adopy –a – Work Unit," : A Model for Safety Improvements., joint commission Journal on quality and safety, February 2004, volume 30, number 2, 59 – 68.

156. AMScanameo, MD, HFillit, MD, "House calls That: a practical guide to seeing the patient home That.," geriatrics That, volume 50, number three, March 1995, 33 – 37.

157. SCSchoenbaum, MD, RRBowbjerg, JD, " malpractice reform must include Steps to Prevent Medical Injury," American College of physicians, 2004 – 53.

158. LChang, MD, "Fibromyalgia a 'Real Disease,' Study Shows," WebMD, http://www.webmd.com/fibromyalgia/news/20081103/fibromyalgia-a-real-disease-study-s.

159. MFreedman,DC, "Fibromyalgia, Chronic Fatigue Syndrome & Hyperbaric Oxygen Therapy," Uncatagorized Comments, 2009.

160. S. Kierstyn, RN DC, "Fibromyalgia vs Parasites, A symptom comparison study, 2002.

161. "Vertebral Subluxation in Chiropractic Practice.," Council on chiropractic practice, clinical practice guideline, number 1, 1998.

162. MWakefield, PhD, RN, " patient safety And Medical Errors, the Journal of legal medicine, that, 23:43 -- 56, 2002.

163. PBarach, MD, MPh, "The End of the Beginning patient safety movement.," Journal of legal medicine, that, 24:7 -- 27, 2003.

164. EErnst, MD, PhD, "chiropractic care: Attempting a Risk Benefit Analysis.": American Journal of Public Health, October, 2002, volume 92, number 10, 1603 – 1611.

165. JLazarou, MSc, HPomeranz, MD< PHD, PNCorey,PhD, "Incidence of Adverse Reactions in Hospitalized Patients."; Journal of the American Medical Association, April 15, 1996, volume 279, number 15 1200 – 1205.

166. CHadida, DC, MRajwani, DC, "It till Your Resumes: case report. Close quotes, Journal of the Canadian chiropractic Association, 1998:42 (four). 216 – 219.

167. DMEisenberg, MD, "Advising Patients Who Seek Alternative Medical Therapies.," annals of internal medicine, volume 127, number 1, 1997, 61 – 69.

168. SHaldeman, MD, DC,m SMRubenstein, DC, "Caught Equine a Syndrome in Patients Undergoing Manipulation of the Lumbar Spine.," spine, that, volume 17, number 12, 1992, 1469 – 1473.

169. ACCLee, BSE, DHLI, MD, DJ Kemper, MD, "chiropractic care for children ," archives of pediatric and adolescent medicine, volume 154, April 2000, 401 – 406.

170. JPattijn, "Complications in Manual Medicine: a review of the literature ," Journal of manual medicine, (1991) 6:89 – 92.

171. MGatterman, DC, "Contraindications and Complications of Spinal Manipulative Therapy," the ACA Journal of chiropractic, September 1981, volume 15, S - 75, 311 – 320.

172. "Recommended Clinical Protocols and Guidelines for the Practice of Chiropractic.," international chiropractic Association That, 2004, http://www.chiropractic.org/Guidelines.

173. PEGeorge, DC, HTSilverstein, DC, PHD, HWallace, DC,MMarshall, BS, MS, "Identification of the High Risk Pre-Stroke Patient.," The ACA Journal of Chiropractic, March, 1981, volume 15, S. - 26.

174. AGTErrett, T.Ed, "It is More Important to Know When Not to Adjust.," chiropractic technique I. that, volume 2, number one, 1990, 1 – 45.

175. ERCrowther, DC, "Miss Cervical Spine Fractures: the importance of reviewing radiographs in chiropractic practice That.," Journal of manipulative and physiological therapeutics That, volume 18, number one, January, 1995, 29 – 33.

176. LHDiamond, ASKliger, MD, RSGoldman, MD, PMPalevsky,MD, "commentary That: quality improvement Projects: How Do We Protect Patient Rights?," American Journal of medical quality That, volume 19, number one, January/February, 2004, 25 – 29.

177. JWSchmidley, MD< TKoch, MD< "The Non-Cerebrovascular Complications of Chiropractic Manipulation.," Neurology, 34, may, 1984, 684-5.

178. MBuna, DC, WCopghlan, DC, MdGruchy,DC, DWilliams, DC, OZmiywsky,DC, "particles of the Atlas That: a review and clinical perspective That.," Journal of manipulative and physiological therapeutics That, I asked for, December 1984, 261 – 266.

179. JDCAssidy, DC, HWThiel,DC, WHKirkaldy-Willis, MD, "Sign Posture Manipulation for Lumbar Intervertebral Dis-Kearny H. and," Journal of manipulative and physiological therapeutics. I. that, DA.

180. NKlougart, DC., CLeboeuf-Yde, DC, LRSassmussen,DC " Safety in Chiropractic Practice. Part one: the occurrences of cerebrovascular accident after manipulation to the neck and can mark from 1978 to 1988.

181. DAVick, DO, CMCKayDO, CRZengerle DO, " the safety of it... Treatment: Literature. From 1925 to 1993.," Journal of American osteopathic Association, volume 96, number two, very wary 1996, 113 – 115.

182. JBalon,etal, "a random I controlled trial of chiropractic spinal manipulation And Children with Chronic Asthma.," Canadian boreal chiropractic college, American thoracic Society convention, 1997.

183. MGatterman, DC, "A Patient Centered Paradigm: a model for chiropractic education and research Allies that.," Journal of alternative and complementary medicine Allies that, volume 1, number four, 1995, 371 – 386.

184. VISimnad, MD "Onset Painful Opthalmoplegia Following Chiropractic Manipulation of the Neck," Western Journal of medicine, I am 166, issue three, March 1997, 207 – 10.

185. ROPistolese, BSc, "risk assessment of neurological, and/or Vertebral Base or Complications in the Pediatric Chiropractic Patient, Journal of vertebral subluxation can't That, two (two), June, 1998, 77 – 86.

186. NHassel, "Pediatric Cephalgia," Journal of clinical chiropractic pediatrics, international chiropractic Association, http://www.firstsearc.oclc.org/WebZ/FSPage?pagename=sagefullrecord"pagetype=print:en...

187. HIshihara, etal, "Facet Joint Asymmetry Is Radiologic Feature a Lumbar Intervertebral Disc Herniation in Children.," Spine, volume 22, issue 17, September 1997, 2001 – 4.

188. CKThompson, Esq, "how Chiropractic Can Protective Its Children." Journal of the American Chiropractic Association, October, 1995.

189. HVernon, CSMcDermaid,CHaginno, "Systematic Review of Randomized Clinical Trials of Complementary/Alternative Therapies in the Treatment of Tension Type and Cervicogenic Headache," complementary therapies in medicine That (1999). 7, 142 – 155.

190. JMLapp, "Pelvic Stress Fracture: Assessment and Risk Factors.," Journal of Manipulative and Physiological Therapeutics, a 161-4754, January 2000, volume 23, issue 1.

191. DJSchimp, DC, "Atypical Sensory Phenomenon: How to Differentiate Migraine, Seizure, And Transient Ischemic Attack.," Topics in Clinical Chiropractic, volume 10, issue three, 1995.

192. JAlcantara, etal, "Management of the Patient with the Lamina Fracture of the Six Cervical Vertebra and Condiment and Subluxation," Journal of manipulative and physiological therapeutics That, February 97, volume 20, issue 2.

193. DPate, DC, DACBR, "Are You Relating Your Patients for Osteoporosis?," Chiro web.com, March 11, 2004, volume 22, issue 6; http://www.chiroweb.com/archives/22/06/15.html.

194. GMGuebert, DC, TARyan, DC., JLRehberger, DC., "Missed Diagnosis, Manipulative Nightmare: A Case Report and Literature Review.," Journal of the Neuromusculoskeletal System, volume 3, number two, Summer 1995, 92 – 96.

195. MTHaneline, DC, "Chiropractic Manipulation of Cervical Intervertebral Disc Herniation.," Journal of the neuromusculoskeletal system That, volume 9, number seven, Spring, 2001, 13 – 15.

196. S. Haldeman, DC, MD, PhD, "Spinal Manipulative Therapy in Sports Medicine.," clinics and sports medicine's That, volume 5, number two, April 1986 277 – 292.

197. S.Haldeman, DC, MD, PhD, FKohlbeck, DC, "medication assisted spinal manipulation That.," the spine Journal, that, too (2002), 288 – 302.

198. GElderfeld, BSc, MSc, "Cauda Equina Syndromes and Conservative Care: Four Case Reports.," British Journal chiropractic, 1999, volume 3, number 4, 98 – 101.

199. MAPCashly DC, "Sir artery migraine or cerebral vascular accident That?," Journal of Manipulative and Physiological Therapeutics, volume 16 number two, February 1993 112-114.

200. VDabbs, DC., WJLauretti, DC., "A Risk Assessment of Cervical Manipulation Versus NSAIDs For the Treatment of Neck Pain," Journal of manipulative and physiological therapeutics That, volume 18, number eight, October, 1995, 530 – 536.

201. HTheil, "Clinical Governance, Clinical Risk Management and the Chiropractic Profession.," Clinical Chiropractic, (2003) 6, 45 – 48.

202. JAQuon, DC, JDCassidy DC., etal, "lumbar intervertebral disc creation That: Treatment by Rotational Manipulation.," Journal of manipulative and physiological therapeutics That, volume 12, number three, June, 1989, 220 – 227.

203. YKLi, etal, "effect of cervical traction Combined with Rotary Manipulation of Cervical Nucleus Proposes Pressures," Journal of manipulative and physiological therapeutics, February 96, volume 21, issue two, 97 – 101.

204. JWAtchison, "manipulation Efficacy: Upper Body.," Journal of Back in Musculoskeletal Rehabilitation, 15 (2000), 3 – 15.

205. VDyck, "upper cervical instability in down syndrome That: A Case Report.," The Journal of the Canadian Chiropractic Association, volume 25, number two, June, 1981, 67 – 8.

206. CAnrig, DC., "Safety Proofing Your Office.," Dynamic Chiropractic, October 4, 1999, volume 17, issue 21, http://www.chirowesb.com/archives/17/21/03.html.

207. MTHaneline, DC, GLewdovitch, DC., "Cervical Manipulation: The Neurosurgeons Perspective?," Chiro.com, dynamic chiropractic, April 21, 2003, volume 21, issue 9; http://www.chiroweb.com/archives/21/09/14.html.

208. KPLee, MD, WGCarline, MD, etal: "Neurologic Complications Following Chiropractic Manipulation: A Survey of California Neurologists.," American Academy of neurology, that, volume 45 (six), June, 1995, 1213 – 1215.

185

209. JMOrley, DC, PhD, ALRosner, PhD, DRedwood,DC., "A Case Study of Misrepresentation of the Scientific Literature: Recent Reviews of Chiropractic.," Journal of Alternative and Complementary Medicine, volume 7, number one, 2001, 65 – 78.

210. C.Mcmakin, DC, "Treatment of Resistant Myofascial Pain with Microcurrent Using Specific Microcurrent Frequencies Applied with Graphite/Vinyl Gloves.," presented to the American backed society, December 11, 1997.

211. F.Wolfe, JJRasker, "The Symptom Intensity Scale, Fibromyalgia, And the Meaning of Fibromyalgia like Symptoms.," The Journal of Rheumatology, 2006; 33:11, 2291 – 2299.

212. F.Wolfe, "Pain Extent and Diagnosis: development and validation of the regional pain scale In 12,799 Patients with Rheumatic Disease.," The Journal of Rheumatology, 2003; 30: 369 – 378.

213. SGRao, MD, et al, "Understanding the Fibromyalgia Syndrome," 1 -- 38, http://us.mg1.mail.yahoo.com/dc/launch?.rand=7pb6laft8g78c.

214. DStarlanyl, MD, "Fibromyalgia Information for Neurologists," http://www.sover.net/~devstar/neuro.htm.

215. Pamphlet: "The Manual Tender Point Survey.," University of Pittsburgh school of medicine, pain evaluation and treatment Institute.

216. JCLowe, DC, GHoneyman-Lowe, DC , "facilitating the decrease in fibromyalgia pain During Metabolic Rehabilitation: An Essential Role for Soft Tissue Therapies.," Journal of bodywork Work and Movement Therapies, October, 1998.

217. Letter: Paula, "the people that don't have FM and/or MPS," 6/27/01, http://www.tidalweb/com/fms/letter.shtml.

218. ABengtsson, KGHenriksson, "The Muscle in Fibromyalgia,: A Review of Swedish Studies," Journal of rheumatology, 1989; "supplement 19" volume 1, 44-48.

219. R. Bennett, MD., "Physical Fitness and Muscle Metabolism in the Fibromyalgia Syndrome: An Overview.," the Journal of rheumatology That 1989; "supplement 19" volume 14, 28 - 39.

220. Cirriculum Comparison, Wester states Chiropractic College vs. Oregon Health Sciences University, l988-1990;"Fibroblasts Form Body Wide Cellular Network.," HM Langevin, CJ Cornbrooks, DJ Taatjes, pop and Histochemical Chemical Cellular Biology, 2004 July; 122 (one): seven – 15.

221. DAlderman, DO., "Prolonged Therapy for Low Back Pain." Practical Pain Management, may 2007.

222. T.Akamaru, MD, et at, "Adjacent Segment Motion after a Simulated Lumbar Fusion in Different Sagittal Alignments: Biomechanical Analysis.," Spine, July 15, 2003, volume 28, issue 14, 1560 -- 1566 .

223. "Manual stimulation, but not electrical stimulation prior to reconstructive surgery, improve functional recovery after facial nerve injuries in rats.," Emanual sckouras et al., Reconstructive Neurology and Neuroscience, 27, (2009). 237 - 251.

224. "Body talk," Co. biology by a photon Lab, new scientist archives, 23 February 02. HTTP://www.tohtech.ac.jp/~elecs/ca/kobayashilab_hp/NewScientistE.html

225. Sell intelligent," Gunther Albrecht Buehler, PhD.

226. "Static timing changes with microcurrent treatment of fibromyalgia associated with cervical spine trauma.," Caroline R. McMakin, Walter M. Gregory, Terry M. Phillips, Journal of bodywork works and movement therapy, (2005) nine, 169 -- 176.

227. "Disc degeneration, therapy Using Marrow Mesenchymal Cell Transplantation: A Report of Two Case Studies" , Takafumi Yoshikawa, MD, et al, http://coll18.coll18.mail.live.com./mail.PrintShell.aspx?type=messaage&cpids=260fd20e.

228. "Why Fusion Sale and Other Insights from the First National Research Congress.," Author Unknown, first international financial research Congress, Boston, October, 2009.

229. "Communicating about Fascia," HM Langevin, MD, PA Huijing, PHD, International Journal of Therapeutic Massage and Bodywork, volume 2, number four, December 2009.

230. "Developments in the Scientific Understanding of Osteoarthritis.," Stephen B. Abramson, McKundun Attur, http://coll8.w.coll18.coll18.mail.live.com/mail/PrintShell.aspx?type=message&cpids-57240ed4-

231. "Rebounding, Good for the Lymph System," will be will, may/june, line 17, number three, http://www.well-being journal.com/index 2.php? Option =com_content&

232. "Poor Spinal Surgery Outcomes for Chronic Low Back Pain," WorkComp Central!, http://www.worktopCentral.com.

233. "Nerve Function," Spinal Nerve Map, Back Talk Systems, 2007, www.backtalksystems.com.

234. "Fighting Addiction with Chiropractic Care," Dynamic Chiropractor, July 29, 2010, volume 28, page 16.

235. "Race, Care Seeking, And Utilization for Chronic Back and Neck Pain: Population Perspectives," The Journal of Pain, volume 11, number four (April), 2010 pages 343 – 350.

236. "Late Sequela of Whiplash Injury with Dissection of Cervical Arteries," V. Hauser, P. Zangger, Y. Winter, W. Oertel, J. Kesseirin, European Neurology, August 18, 2010, vol 64, No 4, p 214 – 218.

237. "Understanding the Wonder of Wellness and how Your Chiropractor Can help Your Achieve It," C. Anrig, DC, To Your Health, Nov, 2010, pg, 6 - 9.

238. "Hormesis, Adaptive Epigeetic Reorganization, and Implications for Human HElath & Longevity," AM Vaiserman, et al; International Dose-Response Society, (formerly Nonlineariety in Biolgoy, Toxicology & Medicine, U. Massachuetts, 2010.

239. "Exploring the NEuromodulatory Effects of the Vertebral Subluxation and Chiropractic Care":, HH Taylor, K. Holt, B Murphy, Chiropractic Journal of Australia, Vol 40, No 1, March 2010, pg 37 – 43.

240. Overdo$ed America, J. Abramson, MD, Harper-Collins Publishers, 2008.
241. "Steroid Shots Bad for Tennis Elbow Long Term," R. Jamer, MD, MedPage Today,
http://co118w.col118.mail.live.com/mail/PrintMessages.aspx?epids=d2d4c05b-deaa=-11df
242. Why Most Published Research Findings are False," JPA Ioannidis, PLos Medicine, August 2005, Vol. 2, Issue 8, e124.
243. "Minimum acceptable outcomes after lumbar spinal fusion," Carragee EJ, Cheng J. Spine Journal, 2010, Apr; 10(4) 313-20.
244. "Cost Effective Osteopathic Manipulative medicine: a literature review of Cost Effectiveness Analyses for Osteopathic Manipulation Technique:, R Gamber DO, MPH, etal, JAOA, vol 105, No 8, Aug 2005, 357 – 368.
245. Effect of a Single Chiropractiac Adjustment on Divergent Thinking and Creative Output: A Pilot Study, Part I," CS Masarsky & M. Todres-Masarsky, Chiropractic Journal of Australia, Vol 4, No 2, June 2010, 57 – 62.
246. "Changes in the Lumbar Spine of Athletes from Supine to the True-Standing Position in Magnetic Resonance Imagiane, Mauch, MD, et al, Spine, Vol 35, No 9, pp 1002 – 1007.
247. "Fascia: a Missing link in our understanding of the pathology of fibromyalgia," Ginevra L, Liptan, etal, Journal of Bodywork & Movement Therapies, Fol 14, Issue 1, p 3 – 12.
248. "Deaths After Chiropractic, A Review of Published Cases:, E Ernst, Int J Clin Practr, 2010, 4 (10): ``62 – 1165.
249. "10 Facts about Fibromyalgia," Health & Fitness: http://healt.msn.com/health-[topics/pain-manaement/fibromyalgia/articlepage.aspx?cp-do...10/26/2010.
250. PManagement of Chronic Spine-Related Conditions: Consensus Recommendations of a Multidisciplinary Panel, RJ Farabaugh, DC, et al, JMPT, Vol 33, No 7, Sept 2010, 484 – 492.
251. "Mechanobiology & Diseases of Mechanotransduction," D E Ingber, MD, PhD, Annals of Medicien, 2003, 35(8) pp 564 - 77.
252. " Clinical Trials: Discerning Hyper from Substance," TR Fleming, PHD, Annals of Internal Medicine, Sept 2010, Vol 153, No 6, 400 – 408.
253. "The Role o fBack Injury or Trauma in Lumbar Disc Degeneration," Spine, Vol 35, No 21, pp 1925 – 1929.
254. "Risk of Dementia and AD with prior Exosure to NSAIDS in an Elderly Community – based Cohort," JCS Breitner, MD, MPH, etal, Neurology, April 22, 2009.
255. The Whistleblower, Confessions of a Healthcare Hitman, Peter Rost, M.D., Soft Skull Press, Brooklyn, New York, 2006
256. White Coat Black Hat, Carl Elliott, Beacon press, Boston, Massachusetts, 2010
257. "Hi resource use found For Chronic Neck Pain," Nancy Walsh, Mid-Page Today,
258. R DOD's Chiropractic Health Care Program
259. "Curing Fascia," an interview with Luigi Stecco by Massimo Ilari, April 2003.
260. "Nerd Genesis: How to Change Your Brain," T. Perlmutter, M.D., The Huffington Post, November 3, 2010.
http://co118w.co1118.mail.live.com/maikl/P:rkntMessages.aspx?epids=d412a074-e76-11DF...
261. "Pediatric Sports Related Concussions: a Review of the Clinical Management of an Oft- Neglected Population," M. W. Kirkwood, K. O. Yeates,, P. E. Wilson, pediatrics 2006; 117; 1359 – 1371.
262. Chiropractic Physiology, M. T. Morter, Jr, DC, B.E.S.T. Research Inc., 1988.
263. Correlative Urinalysis: The Body Knows Best, M. T. Mortar, Junior, DS, MA, DC, she asked he research Inc., 1987.
264. Clinical Biomechanics of the Spine, A.A. White III, M.M. Panjabi, JB Lippincott company, 1978.
265. The Physiology of the Joints: The Trunk of Vertebral Column, I. A̧. Kapanji, Churchill Livingstone, 1974.
266. "The Role of Back Injury Or Trauma In Lumbar Disc Degeneration," M. J. Hancock,, PhD, et al, Spine: 1 October 2010, volume 35, issue 21, PP. 1925 – 1929.
267. "Second Death in a Patient with Idiopathic Scoliosis,"F. Satoh, MD, PhD, et al, Journal of Clinical Forensic Medicine, 13 (2006), 335 – 338.
268. "The influence Of Intervertebral Disc Shape on the Pathway Of Posterior/Posterior Lateral Partial Herniation ," JP Yates,BSc, et al, Spine, volume 35, number seven, PP 735 -- 739 2010.
269. Letter of Opinion: "Death by Chiropractic: Another Mis-Begotten Review," Anthony L. Rosner, PhD, July 26, 2010.
270. Effects of High Velocity, Low Amplitude Manipulation on catalase activity That In Men with Neck Pain," C. Kolberg, DC, et al, J. MPT, volume 33, number four, 300 – 307.
271. Study says brain trauma Can Mimic Lou Gehrig's Disease," A. Swartz, The New York Times, August 17, 2010, http://www.nytimes.com/2010/08/18/sports/18gehrig.html?
272. "Smoking Marijuana Eases Chronic Neuropathic Pain," F. Lowery, Canadian Medical Association Journal, August 30, 2010; http://co118w.co1118.mail.live.com/mail/InboxLight.aspx?FolderID=00000000-0000-0000.
273. Spinal the Delay Shouldn't Impact Cervical Spine Movement and Fitts Task Performance: A Single Blind Randomized before after Trial," SR Passmore, DC, et al, J. MPT, 2010; 33:189 – 192.
274. "The Effects of Spinal Manipulation On the Efficacy of a Rehabilitation Protocol For Patients with Chronic Neck Pain: A Pilot Study," D. Murphy, PhD, DC, et al, J. MPT, 2010; 33:168 – 177.
275. "Immunohistochemical Demonstration of Nerve Endings In Ilio Lumbar Ligament," E. Kiter, M.D. et al, spine, 2010; 35: E101 -- E104.

276. "Spinal Cutaneous Temperature Modification After Spinal Manipulation and L5," RA Roy, DC etal, J. MPT, 2010; 33:308 – 314.
277. From Good Hand to Boxing Gloves, DJ Berardinelli, Trial Guides, LLC, 2009.
278. "Chronic Whiplash and CentralSensitizatin; an Evaluation of the role of a myofascial trigger oints in paoin modulation," MD Freeman, A Nystrom, C centeno, Journal o fBrachial Plexus and Peripheral Nerve Injury, 2009, 4:2.
279. The Ethics of Touch, BEBenjamin, PHD, C Sohmen-Moe, SMA Inc., 2003.
280. Cranial Sutures, M.G. Pick, DC, DICS, Eastland Press, Seattle Wn, l999.
281. An New Management Model for Treating Structural Based Disorders: Dental Orethopedic and Chiropractic Co-Treatment," AS Chinappi, Jr., DDS, H. Getzoff, DC, JMPT, Vol 17, No. 9, Nov/d l994. (Compendium of Sacro Occipital Technique, Peer-Reviewed Literature l984 – 2000 ppgs167 – 173.)
282. "Visceral Manipulation and te Treatment of Uterine Fibroids: a Case Report," K.Cook, BA, S.A. Rasmussen, DC, ACA Journal of Chiropractic, Vol 29, No. 12, Dec. l992. (Compendium of Sacro Occipital Technique, Peer-Reveiwed Literature l984 – 2000 ppgs 137 – 139.
283. "Chiropractic and the Neuroimmune Connection: A Literature Review," A. Cohn, DC, The Journal of Vertebral Subluxation, September 30, 2008.
284. chiropractic training versus medical training course hour Comparison, http://www.chiro.org/LINKS/ABSTRACTS/Chiropractic_s_Medical_Training.shtml
285. "Sleep Disordered Breathing and Mortality: a Prospective Cohort Study," N. Punjabi, etal, PLoS Medicine, August 2009, volume 6, issue eight.
286. Anatomy Trains, Thomas W. Myers, let Livingstone, 2009

Nutritional

1. Effects of soy diet on inflammation induced primary and secondary hyperalgesia in rats; Borzana, TAllb, Zhaoc, Merers and Rajaa, John Hopkins Univ. Baltimore Md, 8, 2009.
2. Vit C Levels in Plasma May Predict Stroke Risk, C. Vega, MD, Jan. 2008,
3. Newsletter, Innate Choice, to EW.innate choice.com September 2009 1-7.
4. K. J. Melanson, "exercise nutrition for adults older than 40 years," American Journal of lifestyle medicine 2008; two; 285 DOI: 10. 1177\1559827608317770.
5. J.E. Kerstetter, K.O.O'Brien, D> M. Caseria, D.E. Wall, K.L.Insogns, "the impact dietary protein on calcium absorption and kinetic measures of bone turnover in women," the Journal of clinical intro chronology and metabolism, 90 (one): 26 – 31
6. every vitamin book, volume 1, researched and compiled by Dennis Jacobs, 2010
7. the ABCs of vitamins and minerals, Jane Heimlich, Phillips publishing, 1992
8. every vitamin book, volume 2, researched and compiled by Dennis Jacobs, 2010
9. C. Emery, "Mediterranean diet reduces need for diabetic drugs.," med page today, HTTP://www.pitched.com/Endo chronology/diabetes 15764? userid= 72646&impressionI... 9/1/2009.
10. J.J. Cannell, M. Zasloff, CF Garland, R. Scragg, E. Giovannucci, "on the epidemiology of influenza" Virology Journal, , 2008, 5:29,
11. "Healthy diet may boost men's fertility," fertility and stability, May 2000.
12. Pamphlet: "novel formulation of THIAA & Berberine offers selective inhibition of matrix metalloproteinase expression within the extracellular matrix.," functional medicine research Center, 2008, 1-7.
13. C.Vega, MD, "vitamin C levels in plasma May predict stroke risk, American Journal of clinical nutrition, 2008; 87:5 -7, 64 – 69.
14. "Vitamin C intake linked to lower risk for type II diabetes.," archives of internal medicine, 2008; 168:1493 – 1499
15. "vitamin C may be effective against common cold primarily in special populations,," Cochrane database systems review, published online July 18, 2007.
16. M. Yoshida, PhD, PF Jacques, SCD, JB Megs, Md, E.Saltzman, MD, MK Shea, MD C Gundberg PHD, B. Dawson-HUghes, MD, G. Dallal, PHD, SL Booth, PHD, "a fact of vitamin K supplementation on insulin resistance in older men and women, diabetes care 31:2092 -- 2096, volume 31, number 11, November 2008.
17. S. Baker, "chemical used on crops could make you fat."; natural news, December 8, 2008
18. Kim Erickson, "Pycynogenol: health and beauty secret?," better nutrition, April 2007, 28 – 29. Edstrom, FNP; "Anti-estrogenic diet,"
19. N. Gardner-Heav;en, PhD, "nutritional protocols normalizing atypical breast thermal injury," Townsend letter for Drs. and patients, November 2004, 60 – 62
20. S. Kierstyn, RN DC, Minerals, Talk notes, 2008
21. Harding, "sugarcane as lower cholesterol.," American Journal of clinical nutrition, November 2008
22. nutrition therapy, 2004
23. Chaga Mushrooms, http://www.chagatrade.ru/chaga/html
24. cheese: treatment of milk for cheesemaking; dairy sciences and technology,http://www.foodsci.uoguelph.ca/dairyedu/cheese.html
25. S. H. Hobbs, DrPH, "the nutritionist what's really on your plate." At times, September 2005, 26

26. R.Cohen, "quit all dairy in just 10 days," not milk,http://bav106hotmail.msn.com/cgi-bin/getmsg?msg=5EBA9402-F72F-BDI 4/8/2005

27. R. Cohen, "crows needs in high school geometry.," not milk, http://bv106fdhav106hotmailmsn.com/cgi-bin/getmsg?msg=24DIC67-FFD7-4166-B7 five -- 22 – 2005

A. Constantine, "Sweet poison, the story aspartame.," http://members.aol.com/bronia/aspartam.htm

28. F.King, DC ND, "homeopathic relief of arthritic pain, dynamic chiropractor, September 13, 2004, 10 – 12

29. B.Tunick, "the sweetest love of all, choose natural alternative to sugar," vegetarian Times, October 2004, 85 to 88

30. R.Cohen, "soymilk spouse," NOTMILK, http://by5fd.bay5.hotmail.msn.com/cgi-bin/getmsg?msg=MSG1095071628.19start=8122 9/13/2004

31. R.Cohen, "drinking water downstream from the dairy farm.," not milk, http://by5fd.bay5.hotmail.msn.com/cgi-bin/getmsg?msg=MSG1094818966.6start=10522..9/10/2004

32. R.Djndaroz et al, "analysis of DNA damage using the comet assay in infants fed cow's milk" Biol Neonate, 2003:84(2)135-41

33. R.Cohen, "Death by Protein," NOTMILK, 8/20/2004

34. Booklet: "new concepts in Lyme disease for chiropractors," focus, allergy research group newsletter, February 2004

35. Opinion Paper: The Nugent Toxin Report, http://www.studentsforlife.net/NugentToxinReport.html

36. K.Bone, "taking the mystery out of fibromyalgia, one herb at a time.," Dr. Jonathan V. Wrights nutrition and healing newsletter, volume 11, issue 7, August 2004

37. R.Harrison, "understanding autoimmune diseases," getting healthy again.com, http://www.gethealthyagain.com/autoimmune.html

38. G. Anderson, "alternative sweeteners, part two," dynamic chiropractic, August 16, 2004, 28,49

39. HJ Roberts, MD, "NutraSweet is a neurotoxin," blatant propaganda article: http://users.actweb.net/~eye/propaganda/articles/aspartame.html

40. JS Turner, "the aspartame/sweet fiasco, Stevia.net; http://www.stevia.net/aparta

41. "safety studies," Stevia.net; http://www.stevia.net/safety.htm

42. "history abuse," Stevia.net; http://www.stevia.net/histor.htm

43. "warning! NutraSweet is a neurotoxin!," the juice guy; http://www.juiceguy.com/NUtrasweet-causes-reduced-sperm-count-shtml

44. RC Cohen, "Summer is for teens and sits," Not Milk, http://by5fd.abay5.hotmail.msn.com/cgi-bin/getmsg?msg=MSG1094908295.6&start=10018..9/14/2004

45. J.V.Wright, MD, "best male antiaging to hold the experts don't want you to have" nutrition and healing, volume 11, issue three, March 2004

46. R.Cohen, "Soy as cancer therapy,"NOTMILK , July 28, 2004

47. R.Cohen, "consuming and protein increases cancer risk.," not no, July 29, 2004

48. J. Mercola, MD, "valuable insights into the importance of vitamin D and son.," http://www.mercola.com/2004/apr/3/vitamin_d_grant.htm

49. "Dr. Linus Pauling unified theory of cardiovascular disease.," the vitamin foundation, http://www.vitaminfoundation.org/unified.htm , 2004

50. O.R. Fonorow, ND, PhD, "theory, history and treatment.," the vitamin C foundation, http://www.thecureforheartdisease.comowen/HeartCure/htm. 2005

51. RF Cathcart III, "a unique function for a score of eight," medical hypotheses; May, 1991:35:32 -- 37

52. J.Mercola, ND, "iron imbalance linked to Parkinson's," http://www.mercola.com/2004/oct/30/iron_imbalance.htm

53. CDC Summary: "introducing the new childhood lead screening questionnaire.," July 27, 2004, volume 53, number 15.

54. D Williams, ND, "the clotbusting miracle that I'm clogs arteries, reverses heart disease.," alternative for the health-conscious individual, Summer 2004, volume 9, number 30

55. RE Holsworth, JR, DO., "Nattokinase and cardiovascular health," Speical Report, 2002.

56. JV Wright, "you're just 24 hours discovering -- and reducing -- your breast cancer risk.," nutrition and healing, volume 10, issue six, July 2003

57. R. Shi, H. Yu, J. McLarty, J Glass, "IGF-I and breast cancer: a meta-analysis": Feist Wheeler Cancer Center, Louisiana State University health sciences Center, Shreveport Louisiana, 71130 -- 3932 USA

58. Suguman, YC Liu, Q. Xia, YS Koh, K. Matsuo, "insulin like factor (IGF) -- one and IGF-I binding protein three and the risk of premenopausal breast cancer: a meta-analysis of literature.," international Journal of cancer, 2004 August 20; 111 (two): 293 – 7

59. JMercola, MD, "antidepressant drugs linked to abnormal bleeding.," http://www.mercola.com/2004/dec/18/antidepressant_drugs.htm

60. JMercola, MD, "the truth about Soy," http://www.mercola.com/2004/dec/4/soy_truth.htm

61. Mercola, MD, "the shadow of Soy," http://www.mercola.com/2003/apr/5/soy_shadow.htm

62. JMercola, MD, "newest research on why you should avoid soy.," http://www.mercola.com/artaicle/soy/avoid_soy.htm

63. M.Adams, "milk products cause Crohn's disease, mucus and irritable bowel syndrome -- interview with Robert Cohen," News Network, http://www.newstarget.com/002684.htm

189

64. R. A. Cohen, Milk, The Deadly Poison, (get info and new copy of book)
65. L.Smeeth, PHD, SL Thomas, PhD, AJHall, PhD, RHUbbard, DM, PFarrington, PhD, PVallance, MD, "risk of myocardial infarction and stroke after infection or vaccination.," New England Journal of Medicine, volume 351:2611 -- 2618
66. JMercola, MD, "flaxseed oil actually increases prostate Cancer, while fish oil decreases it," http://www.mercola.com/2004/jul/21/flax_seed_oil.htm
67. JMercola, MD, "effects of hormone suppression on men with prostate cancer.," http://www.mercola.com/2005/jan/26/hormone_suppression.htm
68. JVWright, MD, "kill the bugs for those that seem less piracy fighters.," Nutrition and Healing, volume 11, issue 11, December 2
69. R.Schultze, ND, "Schultz's five day liver/gall bladder cleansing in the publication program.," http://www.herbdoc.com/p34.asp
70. DGWilliams, ND, "cancer in it can.," Alternative for the Health-Conscious Individual, volume 10 number 11, August 2004, 105 – 109
71. S.Chrubasik, MD, E Eisenberg,MD, EBalan,MD, TWeinberger, MD, RLuzzati, MD, C.Conradt, PHD, "treatment of low back pain exacerbations with willow bark extract: a randomized double-blind study.," the American Journal of medicine, volume 109, number one, July 2000, 9-15
72. R.Cohen, : "Crohn's disease treatment update, 2005" , http://by5fd,bay5.hotmail.msn.com/cgi-bin/getmsg?msg=MSG1110023153.13&start=55680
73. JMercola, MD, Dr. Cole is total health program: hundred and 50 delicious grain free recipes and the proven metabolic type plan to prevent disease, optimize weight And Live Longer, chapter 2.
74. GMHalpern, "anti-inflammatory effects of a stabilized lipid extract of Perna Canaliculus," allergies and immunology's (Paris). 2000 September; 32 (seven): 272-8
75. RCohen, PhD, "terrible twos syndrome," Not Milk, http://by206fd.bay.106.hotmail.msn.com/cgi-bin/getmsg?msg=2D2BF53B-CBB8-4C3199
76. SJOlsen, MYing, MFDavis, MDeasy,BHolland, LLampietro, etal, "multidrug-resistant Salmonella Typhi-murium infection from milk contaminated after pasteurization" Emerg Infect Dis, 2004 May, http://www.cdc.gov.ncidod/FID/vollOno5/03-0484.htm
77. JMeschino,DC, MS, "Polycosanol (saccharum officinarum): an effective natural supplement to lower choles-terol." Dynamic chiropractic, November 18, 2004, 22
78. B.Milor, ELS, "NHS pies, cinnamon, improves glucose and lipid levels.," NNFA today Allies that, volume 18, number 9, September 2004
79. RCohen, "is milk addictive," Not Milk, http://by106fd.bay106.hotmail.msn.com/cgi-bein/getmsg?msg=ACDEE73B-CAOE-481D-B
80. RCohen, "do you require an oil change?," Not Milk, http://by106fd.bay.106hotmail.msn.com/cgi-bin/getmsg?msg=EE504437-E72C-4770.8660
81. "red Clover," Red Clover, http://www.innvistacom/health/herbs/redclove.htm
82. "Pau D'Arco," PauDArco, http://www.innvista.com/health/herbs/paudarco.htm
83. "Ashvagandha" (winter cherry) , Ashvandha, http://www.wrc.net/phyto/Ashvagandha.html
84. "Astralagus," Astralagus, http://www.innvista.com/**health**/herbs/astralag.htm
85. R.Schultze, ND, "the average American's future: diapers and dialysis," Update, October 2003
86. "Saw Palmetto," Whole Health, http://www.health-pages.cm/sp/
87. R. Cohen, "milk and prostate cancer.," Not Milk, April 23, 2004
88. JVWright, MD, "one program, two months, lasting relief -- from almost any symptoms. And the Older You Are, the Better It Works," Nutrition and Healing, volume 11, issue seven, July 2004, 3-8
89. JVWright, MD, "today, and taking injections: which ones were, which was one, and one of the treatments to try first.," Nutrition and Healing, volume 11, issue two, February 2004 1-8
90. JVWright, MD, "sweat your way to a healthier heart -- and a better sex life -- in four weeks or less.," Nutri-tion and Healing, volume 10 issue 12, DC for 2003,
91. J.Wallach, DVM, ND, "the missing 30 minutes of dead doctors don't lie," http://www.american-longevity.com/30min.htm
92. MSJhon, PhD, The Water Puzzle in the Hexagonal Key , uplifting press, Inc., 2004
93. commentary: "spontaneous cervical artery dissections And Implications for Homocysteine," Journal of manipulative physiologic therapeutics, 2004:27:124 – 32;
94. "Water, Our Thirsty World," National Geographic, April, 2010
95. REGrimble, "Immunomodulatory Impact of Dietary Lipids,," Clinical Nutrition Highlights, 2007, Vol 3, Issue 1, 2 - 18
96. JKordich, The Juice Man's Power of Juicing, Wm & Morrow & Co., 1992
97. CAmbridge, Smoothies & Juices. Paragon Publishing, 2003
98. MMWolfe, MD< DR Lichtenstein, MD< GSingh, MD, " gastrointestinal toxicity Of Nonsteroidal Anti-Inflammatory Drugs, New England Journal Of Medicine, June 17, 1999, E. 1888 – 1899
99. C.Anrig, DC., "The Case against Casein.," Chiropractic; March 20, 2000, 20+;
100. JLMayo MD, "Remarkable Health Benefits Of Silly Isoflavones.," clinical nutrition insights That, 1998, volume 6, number 13

101. JCWaterhouse, PhD., "Guaifenesin and a Hypoglycemia Diet in Fibromyalgia" 7/22/02 2002, Http://members.aol.com/SynergyHN/21f.html
102. LMarks, "Fibromyalgia, Herbal Help," 2002
103. JSVolek, RDFeinman, "Carbohydrate Restriction Improves the Features of Metabolic Syndrome. Metabolic Syndrome May Be Defined by the Responses to Carbohydrate Restriction.," Nutrition and Metabolism, 2005, 2:31, 1 – 17
104. MPercival, MD, "Fibromyalgia: Nutritional Support," Clincal Nutrition Insights, 1997.
105. W.Wong, ND, PhD., "Is Fibromyalgia Real," opinion/fact letter, 2004
106. W.Wong, ND., PhD, "Fibromyalgia: Alleviating Its Depression, Sleep Disorders and Overeating,," opinions/fact letter, 2004
107. J.Whitaker, MD, "this cholesterol really matter." Health and healing, 3/15/2010; http: www.naturalnews.com/z028389_cholesterol_health.html

108. J.Whitaker, MD, "Statin Adverse Effects," Health and Healing http://www.statineffects.com/info/adverse_effects.htm
109. "Agency suggests limits on antibiotics in animals, because it rises in drug-resistant bacteria.," http://www.webmd.com/food/recipes/news/20100628/FDA -antibiotics-in-livestock-affects-h...
110. "new review Endorses CD Benefits of Fish Oil.," Lisa Nainggolan, http://www.coll18.coll18.mail.live.com/mail/PrintShell.aspx?type=message&cpids=57903eld-...
111. "S erum B Vitamin Levels and the Risk of Cancer," Journal of the American Medical Association, June 16, 2010, volume 303, number 23, 2377 – 2385
112. "Gary Null & Vit D Toxicity," John Cnanell, MD., Vitamin D newsletter, August 5, 2010.
113. Natural cures "they" don't want you to know about, Kevin Trudeau, aligns publishing group, 2004
114. More Natural "Cures" Revealed, Kevin Trudeau, Alliance Publishing Group, Inc., 2006
115. "more bad news for so a naysayers," Robert A. Cohen, HTTT://health.groups.yahoo.com/group/not milk/message/2953
116. "Reduced Levels of Anti-Inflammatory Cytokines in Patients with Chronic Widespread Pain" , Arthritis and Rheumatism, 2006; 54 (8): 2656 – 2664
117. Rare Earths, Forbidden Cures. Joel D. Wallach, BS, DVM, ND, Ma Lan, MD, MS, DoubleHappiness Publishing Co., POB 1222, Bonita, Ca., 91908, 1994

Glossary of Terms

Adipose tissue: fatty parts of the body; a layer of tissue normally found under the skin in most human, now known to be part of the fascia components of the body, containing a large, body-wide, network of nerve tracts, directing actions and responses of the body's nervous system. Newly recognized, the geography of this network is still under discovery.

Avascular: without cardiovascular vessels (arteries or veins); cartilage contained in vertebral discs is an example of this type of tissue.

Biomechanical: the application of mechanical forces to living organisms. This includes forces that rise from within and outside the body.

Cerebrospinal Fluid: (CSF): a nourishing water cushion, contained within the dura mater, protecting the brain and spinal cord from physical impact.

Dura: (Dura mater): the fibrous membrane forming the outermost of the three coverings of the brain and spinal cord.

Homeostasis: the tendency toward a relatively stable equilibrium between interdependent elements, especially as maintained by physiological processes.

Innate: existing in or belonging to at birth; belonging to the essential nature of something. Also known as innate intelligence.

Metabolism: the sum of the physical and chemical processes in an organism by which its material substance is produced, maintained and destroyed and by which energy is made available; any basic process of organ functioning or operating; all energy and material transformations that occur within living cells.

Neurological: of the nature of a nerve or nerve function.

Organelles: microscopic organs responsible for parts of the cell's activity of self-duplication. Some of the actions produced by these 'body factories' include the duplication of DNA as well as the production of energy molecules.

Organic: pertaining to an organ or of the nature of an organ; of a plant nature vs. a non-plant nature.

Osmosis: the passage of solvent through a semi-permeable membrane separating solutions of different concentrations. The action that allows dense cartilage to 'soak up' its nutrients from the surrounding tissues, assuming, of course, that those tissues are saturated with nutrients.

Physiological: concerning body function or functioning

Physiology: the science of the living organism and its components along with the chemical and physical processes involved.

Somatic: pertaining to the non-reproductive cells or tissues; pertaining to skeletal structures of the body as opposed to visceral/organ structures of the body or the structures associated with the viscera/organs such as visceral muscles.

Synergistically: acting together to and for mutual benefit

Synergism: the harmonious action of two agents, such as drugs or organs, producing an effect that neither could produce alone or an effect that is greater than the total effects of each agent operating by itself.

Syndrome: the sum of the signs and symptoms associated with any pathological process; a group of signs and symptoms that collectively characterize or indicate a particular disease or abnormal condition(s).

About the Author
~ *Sunny Kierstyn RN, DC* ~

Dr. Kierstyn is a *'come up through the ranks'* kinds of doc. Her career path was decided at the age of 4, when she declared one afternoon shortly after her tonsillectomy: "I know: I'll be a nurse!" After that, everything she did was geared toward that goal.

Winning a scholarship in 1960 from Wm. S. Hart High School in Newhall, California enabled her to attend Los Angeles County General Hospital School of Nursing (now known as USC Medical Center). Over the next ten years she became licensed as a Licensed Vocational Nurse (LVN), started a family and earned a degree as a Registered Nurse.

Over the next two decades, her nursing career included service as an Emergency Room RN (Hillside Hospital, San Diego, CA), Operating Room RN (Verdugo Hills Hospital, Glendale, CA, Huntington Memorial Hospital, Pasadena, CA), and at every level of Intensive Care Units (Cedar-Sinai Hospital, Los Angeles, CA), where they have seven busy care units!

Acute-care traditional-western-medicine bedside nursing provided a wonderful base for branching into Chiropractic care. Since graduating in 1989 from Cleveland Chiropractic College in Los Angeles, Dr. Kierstyn has been helping people get out of pain and back into their lives. She established her private practice in Eugene Oregon in 1997, with the addition of the Fibromyalgia Care Center of Oregon in 1999. Serving many people in her community, Dr. Kierstyn's understanding of the human body continues to expand and grow each day.

Choosing chiropractic as a career has been "the most rewarding thing I could ever do," she says. Helping people to get out of pain, to stay out of pain and to walk a path to health is her avid passion. Service in the acute care areas allowed her to understand how many times correction of structural concerns decreases pain patterns without drugs. As a Chiropractic Physician, she witnesses the disease process of many of her patients downtrend and slow (and sometimes stop) when their nerve flow and metabolic flow improve as a result of chiropractic care. She has become very aware of how often-appropriate structural care stops disease problems dead in their tracks.

Discovering – and becoming skilled with – the different possibilities of the broad-scoped Sacral Occipital Technique has provided Dr. Kierstyn a major war-chest full of abilities for addressing the myriad of problems expressed by the American human body. She knows that each condition encompasses the entire body from the spine to the pelvis to the cranium to the abdominal organs themselves.

ALL of it may need attention in order for ALL of it to be healthy. And THAT is what Dr. Kierstyn does: she pays attention to ALL of it!

INTERNATIONAL HEALTH PUBLISHING

Inspiring readers of the world to experience the light.
International Health Publishing books express truth and wisdom,
encourage spiritual enlightenment, facilitate growth and healing –
while also providing a phenomenal reading experience.

International Health Publishing's vision is to increase the number and quality of books and resources available to the public, students and Doctors of Chiropractic – allowing for greater understanding, increased education, as well as more visibility and accessibility of the Chiropractic profession as a means of preventative and continued health care.

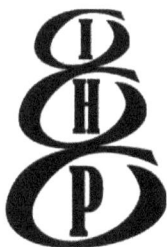

INTERNATIONAL HEALTH PUBLISHING
Adjusting and Growing
International Headquarters • Carrollton, Texas

www.InternationalHealthPublishing.com

www.ingramcontent.com/pod-product-compliance
Lightning Source LLC
Chambersburg PA
CBHW070911270326
41927CB00011B/2530